Onychomycosis

Forthcoming titles in the Series in Dermatological Treatment

Ronald Marks
Facial Skin Disorders

Sakari Reitamo, Thomas Luger and Martin Steinhof
Textbook of Atopic Dermatitis

Onychomycosis
The current approach to diagnosis and therapy

Second edition

Robert Baran MD
Nail Disease Centre, Cannes, France

Roderick Hay MD
Faculty of Medicine and Health Sciences, Queen's University, Belfast, Northern Ireland, UK

Eckart Haneke MD
Dermatology Clinic, Freiburg, Germany

Antonella Tosti MD
Department of Dermatology, University of Bologna, Bologna, Italy

© 1999, 2006 Taylor & Francis, an imprint of the Taylor & Francis Group
Taylor & Francis is the Academic Division of Informa plc

First published in the United Kingdom in 1999 by Martin Dunitz

Second edition published in 2006 by Taylor & Francis, an imprint of the Taylor & Francis Group, 2 Park Square, Milton Park, Abingdon, Oxon OX14 4RN

Tel.:   +44 (0)20 7017 6000
Fax.:   +44 (0)20 7017 6699
E-mail: info.medicine@tandf.co.uk
Website: www.tandf.co.uk/medicine

Although every effort has been made to ensure that drug doses and other information are presented accurately in this publication, the ultimate responsibility rests with the prescribing physician. Neither the publishers nor the authors can be held responsible for errors or for any consequences arising from the use of information contained herein. For detailed prescribing information or instructions on the use of any product or procedure discussed herein, please consult the prescribing information or instructional material issued by the manufacturer.

A CIP record for this book is available from the British Library.

Library of Congress Cataloging-in-Publication Data

Data available on application

ISBN 0-415-38579-2
ISBN 978-0-415-38579-4

Distributed in North and South America by

Taylor & Francis
2000 NW Corporate Blvd
Boca Raton, FL 33431, USA

Within Continental USA
Tel: 800 272 7737;   Fax: 800 374 3401
Outside Continental USA
Tel: 561 994 0555;   Fax: 561 361 6018
E-mail: orders@crcpress.com

Distributed in the rest of the world by
Thomson Publishing Services
Cheriton House
North Way
Andover, Hampshire SP10 5BE, UK
Tel.: +44 (0)1264 332424
E-mail: salesorder.tandf@thomsonpublishingservices.co.uk

Composition by J&L Composition, Filey, North Yorkshire

Printed and bound in Great Britain by CPI Bath

Contents

Contributors

Robert Baran MD
Nail Disease Centre
Cannes, France

Roderick Hay MD
Faculty of Medicine and Health Sciences
Queen's University
Belfast, Northern Ireland, UK

Eckart Haneke MD
Dermatology Clinic
Freiburg, Germany

Antonella Tosti MD
Department of Dermatology
University of Bologna
Bologna, Italy

Bianca Maria Piraccini MD
Department of Dermatology
University of Bologna
Bologna, Italy

Preface to the Second Edition

Fungal infections of the nails (onychomycosis) have become a major source of interest since the development of newer and more effective methods of treating this common skin condition that affects all ages and populations. In the past few years an enormous amount of new information has become available, which has increased current knowledge of the epidemiology, pathogenesis, clinical presentation, diagnosis and management of the condition. We have moved from dealing with a condition, which attracted little interest and a reputation for stubborn resistance to treatment, to one where there is scientific and medical progress and a real possibility for a successful outcome of therapy. With this process has come the realization that there is now a clear choice of treatment determined by rational medical assessment.

This book has been written by clinicians for clinicians. It provides a guide to the steps needed to identify and effectively manage the patient with onychomycosis. It extends the previous work in order to meet the needs of a growing population of patients seeking treatment. We hope that this new edition will provide insight into the diagnosis and management of onychomycosis as well as the most important examples of recent progress in the field.

Robert Baran
Roderick Hay
Eckart Haneke
Antonella Tosti
Bianca Maria Piraccini

Preface to the First Edition

This book is written by clinicians for clinicians. In it the authors, who have an abiding interest in all fields of nail pathology, have focused on one of the commonest of nail disorders, onychomycosis. The stepwise approach provides a basis for identifying the most appropriate cost-benefit considerations in the management of fungal nail infection. Consideration of the subject follows a logical path from clinical expression through laboratory diagnosis to therapy. The new classification of the clinical appearances reflects the underlying nail pathology and provides a rational explanation for the pathogenesis and the response to treatment. Compared with the situation ten years ago, there is now a wide choice of treatment options for patients with onychomycosis from topical antifungal agents to nail surgery. The development of new treatment regimens, however, has had the greatest impact on the success of therapy. This in turn has opened the possibility of successful treatment to the majority of patients with fungal nail infections, particularly those caused by dermatophytes. The result has been a major increase in the numbers of patients with onychomycosis presenting for treatment. We hope that this book will provide an up to date review of this common clinical problem which will be of interest to a wide group of health professionals including dermatologists, general practitioners, practice nurses and chiropodists/podiatrists.

The authors

Epidemiology

Onychomycoses are the most common of nail diseases. They occur worldwide, but with variable frequency depending on different climatic, professional and socio-economic conditions. One hundred years ago, they were considered to be very rare, affecting mainly those caring for children with tinea capitis, but their prevalence has increased dramatically during the last few decades (Table 1.1).[1,2]

Approximately 1.5–15% of persons presenting to a dermatologist have an onychomycosis.[3] Other estimates are between 2%[4] and 23%.[5] There are considerable differences in the prevalence: a survey on 20 000 persons from North Malawi found no onychomycosis, although there was a 1.5–2.5% prevalence of dermatophytes in this population;[6] this is probably due to the fact that many of the people do not wear shoes. The frequency of onychomycosis in rural Zaire was 0.89%, but 4% of men and 2.8% of women in towns had fungal nail infections.[7] Large-scale studies from Europe, the Middle East and North

| TABLE 1.1 | Proportion of onychomycoses to dermatomycoses (literature survey; from ref. 1) and increase in prevalence in recent years |

CITY	YEAR	%
Paris	1910	0.2
Munich	1913–1922	0.13
Berlin	1919–1934	2
Munich	1938	2.6
Hamburg	1938	2.8
Hamburg	1949	10
Munich	1951	8.4
Berlin	1951–1956	17.1
Munich	1958	11.1
Brussels	1980	30
Increase in prevalence[2]		10^{-6}
Icelandic children	1985	1.65*
	2000	21.3*

*Prevalence per 100 000.

America revealed very high rates of fungal nail infections (Table 1.2). A prevalence of 27% was found in coal miners; heat, humidity and common shower facilities were held to be responsible for this high proportion.[8] In another study carried out 10 years later, 327 of 1000 persons from the Ruhr area in Germany were found to have a dermatophyte infection of their nails.[9]

The prevalence of onychomycosis appears to parallel that of foot ringworm (Table 1.2).

Onychomycoses increase in frequency with age. Whereas they are very rare in young children – two studies found 0.2%, other studies failed to find a single case, the latest one revealed an overall prevalence of 0.22% in Iceland[2,11–15] – they are common in young adults and very frequent in the elderly.[13] Among adolescents, young males are more frequently affected than females; this is probably due to more frequent nail damage from sports and leisure activities among male adolescents. Several large-scale surveys revealed that approximately 14–18% of the general population have a fungal nail infection, with 48% of people >70 years, and that the increase in prevalence is related to age until about 80 years when the prevalence drops again slightly[16,17] (Table 1.3).[4–9,13–16,18–36]

In all, 18–40% of all nail diseases are fungal infections[37,38] and approximately 30% of all dermatomycoses are mycotic nail infections.[3]

By far the most common pathogens are dermatophytes. Virtually unknown in Western Europe at the beginning of the 20th century, *Trichophyton rubrum* was introduced from West Africa and Asia, and has become the most frequent pathogen in Western Europe, North America, and Asia, with 50–75% of all onychomycoses.[39,40] *T. rubrum* and *T. mentagrophytes* together account for at least 80% of onychomycoses in Central Europe.[41] Yeasts are cultured from 5–17% of these cases, with >70% of these being *Candida albicans*.[42] Non-dermatophyte moulds are considered the pathogen in less than 5%[41,43–46] and even this low number is debatable.[47] *Scytalidium dimidiatum, S. hyalinum* and *Scopulariopsis brevicaulis* are generally accepted as nail pathogens as well as some *Aspergillus, Fusarium* and *Acremonium* spp. and *Onychocola canadensis*.[48] Many non-dermatophyte mould onychomycoses are associated with paronychia.[36] However, there are considerable variations according to geographical location:[49] up to 50% of the onychomycosis cases among Thai conscripts were due to *Scytalidium dimidiatum (Hendersonula toruloidea)*.[50] In Saudi

TABLE 1.2	Prevalence of fungal foot infection[10]
GROUP	PREVALENCE OF FOOT INFECTION (%)
Swimmers	8.5
Day schoolboys	8.9
Boarding schooolboys	22
Male long-stay hospital patients	39
Coal miners	Up to 80%

TABLE 1.3	Prevalence of onychomycoses worldwide			
COUNTRY	YEAR OF PUBLICATION	PREVALENCE (%)	SUBJECTS EXAMINED	REFERENCE NO.
Germany	1965	27	Coal miners	8
Britain	1966	2		4
East Germany	1966	13		5
USA	1972	>15–20	Estimate	11
Germany – Ruhr area	1974	32.7	1000 persons	9
Zaire (Congo)	1977	0.9	Rural areas	7
		2.8	Urban areas – male	
		4	– female	
Great Britain	1992	2.7	Omnibus survey	19
Spain	1995	2.6	Computer-assisted telephone interview system	20
Greece	1995	2.5	Fingernails	21
		11.7	Toenails	
Finland	1995	8.4	All ages	22
		11.3	Adults	
		4.3	Females	
		13	Males	
North Malawi	1996	0	20 000 rural area	6
Great Britain	1996	11	100 non-diabetics	23
USA	1996	50.3	Dermatological patients	24
Italy	1996	24.8	Dermatological patients	25
Hong Kong	1997	14.2	Urban dermatological patients	26
Ontario, Canada	1997	6.9	Dermatological patients	27
Ohio, USA	1997	14	General population	16
Canada & USA	1997	0.44	2500 children and adolescents under 18 years	13
Canada	1997	9.7	Psoriatics	14
Greece	1998	15.7	Dermatological study	15

TABLE 1.3		Prevalence of onychomycoses worldwide (cont)		
COUNTRY	YEAR OF PUBLICATION	PREVALENCE (%)	SUBJECTS EXAMINED	REFERENCE NO.
Turkey	1999	41.2	Mycology study	28
Pakistan	1999	100 of suspected OM	Mycology study	29
Europe	1999	29.6	Dermatology patients	30
		21.1	General practitioners' patients	
Canada–USA	2000	13.8	Patients of one general practitioner	31
Tunisia	2001	67.1	4-year study	32
Brazil	2003	39	2-year study dermatology	33
Mexico	2004	47	Patients over 65 years	34
Paraguay	2005	6	Mycological samples from children	35
Sri Lanka	2005	66	128 onychomycosis-suspected patients	36
Iceland	2005	1.65/10*	1982–1985	2
		21.3*	1996–2000	
		0.22	2000	

*1 : 100 000.

Arabia, most onychomycoses were due to *C. albicans*, with 204 of 243 culturally positive cases of onychomycosis and 241 of 257 cases secondary to paronychia.[51] A Hungarian study showed that as regards nails which had either been negative or grown yeasts, 60% more dermatophytes could be grown after nail avulsion.[52] Further, a certain change in fungal pathogen pattern has been noted during recent decades.[53]

Toenails are about seven times more frequently affected than fingernails. The reason for this was thought to be the growth rate, which is about three times slower for toenails than fingernails.[48] However, it has been repeatedly found that active onychomycosis slows down the growth rate and that this may become normal after cure,[54–57] strongly suggesting that other ageing factors may play a more important role.

The enormous increase in the prevalence of onychomycosis is attributed to various factors. The simplest explanation, although not yet discussed in the literature, is that a contagious disease like superficial dermatomycosis and particularly onychomycosis, that has not been treated sufficiently or at all stands a good chance of spreading. The time curve of the exponential increase in the prevalence fits exactly with this assumption. Genetic susceptibility promotes the increase in prevalence. However, in practice, it may be difficult in a particular case to differentiate environmental from genetic factors.[58] Increased and prolonged exposure to fungal pathogens through communal bathing and showering facilities, ritual washing,[32] health spas, saunas, and gyms, sports activities, wearing occlusive footgear, ageing of the population, increasing numbers of diabetics, administration of immunosuppressive and cytotoxic drugs, and the AIDS epidemic are all thought to enhance the risk of fungal nail infections.[59,60] However, a series of investigations from France showed that although the main fungal pathogen isolated from public sports facilities was *T. mentagrophytes* the fungi isolated from the feet of the users were mostly *T. rubrum*.[61] Another study from Wales also did not support the assumption that frequent use of public changing facilities would be related to the transmission of fungal infection; instead, the high proportion of parents affected suggested that they

might act as the source of infection.[13] English[62] was the first to observe that there was a high risk of intrafamilial onychomycosis infection of the toes, whereas conjugal infection rates were low. Genetic investigations from Italy and France suggest that the susceptibility to fungal nail infections, particularly to *T. rubrum* onychomycosis, might be inherited as an autosomal dominant trait.[63] An examination of more than 18 500 subjects revealed that a familial disposition increases the odds for onychomycosis by a factor of almost 4.[17,64]

Almost all surveys agree that onychomycoses are more prevalent in men than in women, although the differences vary considerably;[65] only one Spanish survey found more onychomycosis in women than in men (1.8% vs. 0.8%).[66] Interestingly, reports from three Muslim countries (Iran, Pakistan and Saudi Arabia) showed more fingernail mycoses in women than in men and a predominance of *C. albicans*.[30,51,67,68]

Damaged nails are more susceptible to onychomycosis.[4,68] This is supported by the observation that dermatophytes can be grown from normal toenails and that dermatophyte onycholysis of the big toenail healed after correction of the underlying foot deformity.[69,70]

Sports activities increase the risk of onychomycosis. On the one hand, this appears to be contradictory, as sports should improve the arterial blood supply to the feet including the toes. On the other hand, sports probably lead to increased foot trauma thus increasing the risk of fungal infection, but a wet environment for swimmers and other persons practising aquatic sports may also play an important role.

Climatic factors play an important role for pathogenic fungi, particularly non-dermatophyte moulds,[36] whereas the increased frequency of *C. albicans* as a cause of onychomycosis in warm climates, particularly in Middle East countries, was recently disputed.[71]

Wearing closed shoes is another factor that renders the feet more susceptible to fungal infection. The humid and warm microclimate favours the growth of pathogenic fungi. A similar situation is found in individuals engaged in professions where they are obliged to wear protective shoes.

Tinea unguium was seen in 42% of subjects with arterial circulatory disorders.[72] More recent studies indicate peripheral arterial disease and smoking as risk factors.[73–75]

Although previous investigations on the role of diabetes mellitus were contradictory[23] it is now accepted that diabetes mellitus increases the risk for onychomycosis – mainly through its effect on microcirculation, rather than immunity.[76–82] The majority of more recent studies found a higher prevalence of onychomycosis in diabetics, by up to one third.[67] One study found an increase in *Candida* infections,[81] but this was not confirmed by other authors.[82] Diabetes mellitus may also be an aggravating factor for other secondary infections and erysipelas.[83–85]

Nail changes alone were seen in 8%, and nail and interdigital changes in an additional 22% of patients with venous abnormalities (controls 4% and 0%, respectively); however, cultures were positive in only 9% of patients and 1% of controls[86,87] (Table 1.4).[4,9,16,23,27,45,78,82,85–91]

Psoriasis apparently increases the risk of acquiring onychomycosis, particularly of the toenails.[27,88,89,92–96] The generally held opinion that onychomycosis would be less frequent in psoriatic nails because dermatophytes do not survive in parakeratotic keratin and, in particular, are not found where there is pronounced exudation of serum and hence serum inclusion in the parakeratosis is not true, as many investigations including some with deep nail biopsies have shown.[96–99]

Hereditary palmoplantar keratoses also appear to favour fungal nail infections.[91]

Immunodeficiencies play a major role in the literature on onychomycoses. It has long been known that severe nail involvement is a virtually mandatory feature of chronic mucocutaneous candidosis.[100–103] Other immunodeficiencies with a higher risk of onychomycosis are organ transplantation,[104–107] Cushing's syndrome and iatrogenic hypercortisolism,[108] and systemic lupus erythematosus.[109]

There is a vast literature on onychomycosis in HIV-positive patients. Up to 30% to almost 78% of AIDS patients are said to have onychomycosis.[110,111] HIV-positive patients may develop a particular form of proximal white subungual onychomycosis, which is almost diagnostic of AIDS.[112,113]

TABLE 1.4	Frequency of onychomycoses and importance of predisposing diseases			
DISEASE	**NUMBER EXAMINED**	**ONYCHOMYCOSIS (%)**		**REFERENCE NO.**
Abnormal toenails	72	43		4
Subungual hyperkeratoses	183	34		4
Podiatric patients	168	37		4
Impaired arterial circulation	112	42		45
Venous insufficiency	100	10 (30)	Culture-proven (altered nails)	86
Venous insufficiency	36	59		87
Diabetes mellitus	100	12		23
Diabetes mellitus	550	. . .	2.7 times more frequent than in matched population and 3 times more frequent in men than in women	78,82
Diabetes mellitus		17%	Vs. 6.8 in non-diabetics	85
Diabetes mellitus type II (with onychomycosis-reminiscent nail changes)	190	65.3		90
Vs. matched controls	190	51.5		
Psoriasis	100	14	Dermatophytes	9
		16	*Candida* spp.	
		16	Moulds	
Psoriasis	120	35	All fungi	88
		24	Dermatophytes	
		15	*Candida albicans*	
Psoriasis	78	27	All nails in psoriatics	89
		23	Normal-appearing nails	
		30	Altered nails	

TABLE 1.4	Frequency of onychomycoses and importance of predisposing diseases (cont)			
DISEASE	NUMBER EXAMINED	ONYCHOMYCOSIS (%)		REFERENCE NO.
Psoriasis	561	13	All nails	27
	298	0.7	Normal-appearing nails	
	263	27	Clinically abnormal nails	
Keratosis palmoplantaris	. . .	. . .		91
Old age (> 70 years)	. . .	48		16

All studies agree that the prevalence of onychomycosis increases with age.[16,17,48,114,115]

References

1. Haneke E. Epidemiology and pathology of onychomycoses. In Nolting S, Korting HC, eds. Onychomycoses. Berlin, Springer, 1989:1–8

2. Sigurgeirsson B, Hilmarsdottir I, Jonasson PS. Onychomycosis in Icelandic children. J Eur Dermatol Venereol; in press

3. Achten G, Wanet-Rouard J. Onychomycosis (Mycology No. 5). Brussels, Cilag, 1981

4. Walshe MM, English MP. Fungi in nails. Br J Dermatol 1966; 78:198–207

5. Seebacher C. Untersuchungen über die Pilzflora kranker und gesunder Zehennägel. Mykosen 1966; 11:893–902

6. Pönninghaus JM, Clayton Y, Warndorff D. The spectrum of dermatophytes in northern Malawi (Africa). Mykosen 1996; 39:293–7

7. Vanbreuseghem R. Prévalence des onychomycoses au Zaïre particulièrement chez les coupeurs de canne à sucre. Ann Soc Belg Med Trop 1977; 57:7–15

8. Götz H, Hantschke D. Einblicke in die Epidemiologie der Dermatomykosen im Kohlenbergbau. Hautarzt 1965, 16:543

9. Götz H, Patiri C, Hantschke D. Das Wachstum von Dermatophyten auf normalem und psoriatischem Nagelkeratin. Mykosen 1974; 17:373–7

10. Roberts DT, Evans EGV, Allen BR. Fungal Infection of the Nail, 2nd edn. London, Mosby-Wolfe, 1998:58

11. Khosravi AR, Aghamirian MR, Mahmoudi M. Dermatophytoses in Iran. Mycoses 1994; 37:43–8

12. Philpot CM, Shuttleworth D. Dermatophyte onychomycosis in children. Clin Exp Dermatol 1989; 14:203–5

13. Gupta AK, Sibbald RG, Lynde CD et al. Onychomycosis in children: prevalence and treatment strategies. J Am Acad Dermatol 1997; 36:395–402

14. Gupta AK, Lynde CW, Jain HC et al. A higher prevalence of onychomycosis in psoriatics compared with non-psoriatics: a multicentre study. Br J Dermatol 1997; 136:786–9

15. Rigopoulos D, Katsiboulas V, Koumantakis E, Emmanouii P, Papanicolaou A, Katsambas A. Epidemiology of onychomycosis in southern Greece. Int J Dermatol 1998; 37:925–8

16. Elewski BE, Charif MA. Prevalence of onychomycosis in patients attending a dermatology clinic in northeastern Ohio for other conditions. Arch Dermatol 1997; 133:1172–3

17. Haneke E, Roseeuw D. The scope of onychomycosis. Epidemiology and clinical features. Int J Dermatol 1999; 38 Suppl 2:7–12

18. Zaias N. Onychomycosis. Arch Dermatol 1972; 105:263

19. Roberts DT. Prevalence of dermatophyte onychomycosis in the United Kingdom: results of an omnibus survey. Br J Dermatol 1992; 126 Suppl 39:23–7

20. Sais G, Jucgla A, Peyri J. Prevalence of dermatophyte onychomycosis in Spain: a cross-sectional study. Br J Dermatol 1995; 132:758–61

21. Devliotou-Panagiotidou D, Koussidou-Eremondi T, Badillet G. Dermatophytosis in northern Greece during the decade 1981–1990. Mycoses 1995; 38:151–7

22. Heikkilä H, Stubb S. The prevalence of onychomycosis in Finland. Br J Dermatol 1995; 133:699–703

23. Buxton PK, Milne LJR, Prescott RJ, Proudfoots MC, Stuart FM. The prevalence of dermatophyte infection in well-controlled diabetics and the response to Trichophyton antigens. Br J Dermatol 1996; 134:900–3

24. Kemma ME, Elewski BE. A US epidemiologic survey of superficial fungal diseases. J Am Acad Dermatol 1996; 35:539–42

25. Mercantini R, Marsella, R, Moretto D. Onychomycosis in Rome, Italy. Mycopathologia 1996; 136:25–32

26. Kam KM, Au WF, Wong PY, Cheung MM. Onychomycoses in Hong Kong. Arch Dermatol 1997; 133:1172–3

27. Gupta AK, Jain HC, Lynde CW, Watteel GN, Summerbell RC. Prevalence and epidemiology of unsuspected onychomycosis in patients visiting dermatogists' offices in Ontario, Canada. A multicenter survey of 2001 patients. Int J Dermatol 1997; 36:783–7

28. Kıraz M, Yegenoğlu Y, Erturan Z, Ang O. The epidemiology of onchomycoses in Istanbul, Turkey. Mycoses 1999; 42:323–9

29. Bokhari MA, Hussain I, Jahangir M, Haroon TS, Aman S, Khurshid K. Onychomycosis in Lahore, Pakistan. Int J Dermatol 1999; 38:591–5

30. Abeck D Haneke E, Nolting S, Reinel D, Seebacher C. Onychomykose. Dtsch Ärztebl 2000; 97:A-1984–1986

31. Ghannoum MA, Hajjeh RA, Scher RK et al. A large-scale North American study of fungal isolates from nails: the frequency of onychomycosis, fungal distribution, and antifungal susceptibility patterns. J Am Acad Dermatol 2000; 43:641–8

32. Anane S, Aoun K, Zallagura N, Touratbine A. Onychomycoses dans la région de Tunis. Données épidémiologiques et mycologiques. Ann Dermatol Venereol 2001; 128:6–7

33. Aranjo AJG, Bastos OMP, Souza MAJ, Oliveira JC. Occurrence of onychomycosis among patients attended in dermatology offices in the city of Rio de Janeiro, Brazil. An Bras Dermatol 2003; 78:299–308

34. Cedeño L, Vasquez del Mercado E, Arenas R. Onicomicosis en pacientes geriátricos. Datos de 435 casos estudiados en diez años. Dermatol Cosm Méd Quir 2004; 2:236–40

35. Ortiz de Da Silva D, de Lacarruba LF, Guzmán A. Dermatofitosis infantiles in Asunción, Paraguay. Dermatol Cosm Méd Quir 2005; 3:22–6

36. Ranawaka RR, Rasgunathan RW, De Silva N. Epidemiology and clinical features of onychomycosis in Sri Lanka (A study done in Galle district on 128 patients). Sri Lanka Ass Dermatol Ann Meet & Joint Meet German Dermatol Soc, 24–27 Feb 2005, Colombo – Kandy, Book Abstr 2005:18

37. Langer H. Epidemiologische und klinische Untersuchungen bei Onychomykosen. Arch Klin Exp Dermatol 1957; 204:624

38. Achten G, Wanet-Rouard J. Onychomycoses in the laboratory. Mykosen 1978; 23 Suppl 1:125

39. Dardé ML. Epidémiologie des dermatophyties. Ann Dermatol Venereol 1992; 119:99–100

40. Manzano-Gayosso P, Méndez-Tovar LJ, Hernández-Hernández F, López-Martínez R. Dermatophytoses in Mexico City. Mycoses 1994; 37:49–52

41. Clayton YM. Clinical and mycological diagnostic aspects of onychomycoses and dermatomycoses. Clin Exp Dermatol 1992; 17 Suppl 1:37–40

42. Cohen J, Scher RK, Pappert A. The nail and fungus infections. In Elewski B, ed. Cutaneous Fungal Infections. New York, Igaku Shoin, 1992:106–23

43. Summerbell RC, Kane J, Krajden S. Onychomycosis, tinea pedis, and tinea manuum caused by non-dermatophytic filamentous fungi. Mycoses 1989; 32:609–19

44. Willemsen MD. Changing pattern in superficial infections: focus on onychomycosis. J Eur Acad Dermatol Venereol 1993; 2:S6–S11

45. Williams HC. The epidemiology of onychomycosis in Britain. Br J Dermatol 1993; 129:101–9

46. Greer DL. Evolving role of nondermatophytes in onychomycosis. Int J Dermatol 1995; 34:521–34.

47. Ellis DH, Watson AB, Marley JE, Williams TG. Non-dermatophytes in onychomycosis of the toenails. Br J Dermatol 1997; 136:490–3

48. Haneke E. Fungal infections of the nail. Semin Dermatol 1991; 10:41–53

49. Elewski BE, Hay RJ. Update on the management of onychomycosis: Highlights of the Third Annual International Summit on Cutaneous Antifungal Therapy. Clin Infect Dis 1996; 23:305–13

50. Kotrajaras R, Chongsathein S, Rojanavanich V, Buddhavudhikarai P, Viriyayadhakorn S. Hendersonula toruloidea infection in Thailand. Int J Dermatol 1988; 27:391–5

51. Al-Sogair SM, Moawad MK, Al-Humaidan YM. Fungal infection as a cause of skin disease in the Eastern Province of Saudi Arabia: prevailing fungi and pattern of infection. Mycoses 1991; 34:333–7

52. Szili M, Sándor L. Comparative mycological studies from nails removed because of onychomycosis. Börgyógy Venerol Szle 1984; 60:175–7 (in Hungarian)

53. Ginter G, Rieger E, Heigl K, Propst E. Steigende Häufigkeit der Onychomykose – Ändert sich das Erregerspektrum? Mycoses 1996; 39 Suppl 1:118–22

54. Na GY, Suh YO, Choi SK. A decreased growth rate of the toenail observed in patients with distal subungual onychomycosis. Ann Dermatol 1995; 7:217–21

55. De Berker D, Angus B. Proliferative compartments in the normal nail unit. Br J Dermatol 1996; 135:555–9

56. Goulden V, Goodfield MJ. Onychomycosis and linear nail growth. Br J Dermatol 1997; 136:139–40

57. Yu HJ, Kwon HM, Oh DH, Kim JS. Is slow nail growth a risk factor for onychomycosis? Clin Exp Dermatol 2004; 29:415–18

58. Evans EGV. Causative pathogens in onychomycosis and the possibility of treatment resistance: a review. J Am Acad Dermatol 1998; 38:S32–S36

59. Barranco V. New approaches to the diagnosis and management of onychomycosis. Int J Dermatol 1994; 33:292–9

60. Conant MA. The AIDS epidemic. J Am Acad Dermatol 1994; 31 Suppl:S47–S50

61. Feuilhade M. Pied et mycoses. Aspects épidémiologiques. Pied 1990; 6:5–6

62. English MP. *Trichophyton rubrum* infections in families. Br Med J 1957; 2:744–6

63. Zaias N, Tosti A, Rebell G et al. Autosomal dominant pattern of distal subungual onychomycosis caused by *Trichophyton rubrum*. J Am Acad Dermatol 1996; 34:302–4

64. Burzykowski T, Molenberghs G, Abeck D et al. High prevalence of foot diseases in Europe: results of the Achilles project. Mycoses 2003; 46:496–505

65. Roseeuw D. Achilles foot screening project: preliminary results of patients sreened by dermatologists. J Eur Acad Dermatol Venereol 1999; 12 Suppl 1:S6–S9

66. Velez A, Diaz F. Onychomycosis due to saprophytic fungi. Report of 25 cases. Mycopathologia 1985; 91:87–92

67. Chabasse D. Epidémiologie et étiologie des onychomycoses. In Baran R, Piérard GE. Onychomycoses. Paris, Masson, 2004:1–35

68. Male O, Tappeiner J. Nagelveränderungen durch Schimmelpilze. Dermatol Wschr 1965; 151:212–21

69. Baran R, Badillet G. Un dermatophyt unguéal est-il nécessairement pathogène? Ann Dermatol Venererol 1983; 110:629–31

70. Baran R, Badillet G. Primary onycholysis of the big toenail: a review of 112 cases. Br J Dermatol 1982; 106:529–34 (abstract)

71. Evans EGV. Causative pathogens of onychomycosis in warm climates. J Eur Acad Dermatol Venereol 2002; 16 Suppl 1:216

72. Dahlke H. Zur Pathogenese der Tinea pedis, insbesondere bei peripheren Durchblutungsstörungen. Mykosen 1971; 14:409–13

73. Rodriguez-Soto ME, Fernandez-Andreu CM, Moya Duque S, Rodriguez Diaz RM, Martinez-Machin G. Clinico-mycological study of onychomycosis in elderly patients. Rev Inst Med Trop São Paulo 1993; 35:213–17

74. Scher RK. Onychomycosis is more than a cosmetic problem. Br J Dermatol 1994; 130 Suppl:15

75. Gupta AK, Gupta MA, Summerbell RC et al. The epidemiology of onychomycosis: possible role of smoking and arterial disease. J Eur Acad Dermatol Venereol 2000; 14:466–9

76. Evans SL, Nixon BP, Lee I, Lee D, Mooradian AD. The prevalence and nature of podiatric problems in elderly diabetic patients. J Am Geriatr Soc 1991; 39:241–5

77. Alteras I, Saryt E. Prevalence of dermatophytosis in patients with diabetes. J Am Acad Dermatol 1992; 26:408–10

78. Gupta AK, Humke S. The prevalence and management of onychomycosis in diabetic patients. Eur J Dermatol 2000; 10:379–84

79. Romano, C, Massai L, Asta F, Signorini AM. Prevalence of dermatophytic skin and nail infections in diabetic patients. Mycoses 2001; 44:85–6

80. Lugo-Somolinos A, Sanchez JL. Prevalence of dermatophytosis in patients with diabetes. J Am Acad Dermatol 1992; 26:408–10

81. Rich P. Special patient populations: onychomycosis in the diabetic patient. J Am Acad Dermatol 1996; 35:S10–S12

82. Gupta AK, Konnikov N, MacDonald P et al. Prevalence and epidemiology of toenail onychomycosis in diabetic subjects: a multicenter survey. Br J Dermatol 1998; 139:665–71

83. Girmenia C, Arcese N, Micozzi A. Onychomycosis as a possible origin of disseminated *Fusarium* spp infection in a patient with severe aplastic anemia. Clin Infect Dis 1992; 14:1167

84. Badillet G. Dermatophyties et Dermatophytes. Paris, Ed Varis, 1990:303

85. Dogra S, Kumar B, Anil B, Bhansali A, Chakrabarty A. Epidemiology of onychomycosis patients with diabetes mellitus in India. Int J Dermatol 2002; 412:647–51

86. Wienert V, Stemmer R. Onychomykosen bei phlebologischen Patienten. Phlebol Proktol 1982; 11:281–3

87. Del Mar M, De Ocariz S, Arenas R, Ranero-Juarez GA, Farrera-Esponda F, Monroy-Ramos E. Frequency of toenail onychomycosis in patients with cutaneous manifestations of chronic venous insufficiency. Int J Dermatol 2001; 40:18–25

88. Feuerman E, Alteras I, Aryelly J. The incidence of pathogenic fungi in psoriatic nails. Castellania 1976; 4:195–6

89. Staberg B, Gammeltoft MD, Onsberg P. Onychomycosis in patients with psoriasis. Acta Dermatol Venereol 1983; 63:436–8

90. Piérard GE, Piérard-Franchimont C. The nail under fungal siege in patients with type II diabetes mellitus. Mycoses 2005; 48:339–42

91. Nielsen PG, Faergemann J. Dermatophytes and keratin in patients with hereditary palmoplantar keratoderma. Acta Derm Venereol 1993; 73:416–18

92. Fransson J, Stogards K, Hammar H. Palmoplantar lesions in psoriatic patients and their relation to inverse psoriasis, tinea infection and contact allergy. Acta Derma Venereol 1985; 65:218–22

93. Malka N, Contet-Audonnet N, Reichert-Penetrat S, Trucheret F, Barbaud A, Schmutz JL. Onychomycoses et psoriasis unguéal. J Mycol Med 1998; 8:192–5

94. Ständer H, Ständer M, Nolting S. Häufigkeit des Pilzbefalls bei Nagelpsoriasis. Hautarzt 2001; 52:418–22

95. Kjellberg-Rarsen G, Haederstal M, Sejgaard EL. The prevalence of onychomycosis in patients with psoriasis and other skin diseases. Acta Derm Venereol 2003; 83:206–9

96. Haneke E. Nail biopsies in onychomycosis. Mykosen 1985; 28:473–80

97. Haneke E. Bedeutung der Nagelhistologie für die Diagnostik und Therapie der Onychomykosen. Ärztl Kosmetol 1988; 18:248–54

98. Haneke E. Pathogenesis of onychomycoses. Dermatology 1998; 197:200–1

99. Lawry M, Haneke E, Storbeck K, Martin S, Zimmer B, Romano P. Methods for diagnosing onychomycosis: a comparative study and review of the literature. Arch Dermatol 2000; 136:1112–26

100. Haneke E, Djawari D. Hyperimmunglobulin E-Syndrom: Atopisches Ekzem, Eosinophilie, Chemotaxisdefekt, Infektanfälligkeit und chronische mucocutane Candidose. Akt Dermatol 1982; 8:34–9

101. Haneke E, Djawari D. Ketoconazole therapy of chronic mucocutaneous candidosis. In: Baxter M. Proceedings of the VIII Congress of the International Society for Human and Animal Mycology. Palmerston North, Massey University Press, 1983

102. Hay RJ, Baran R, Moore MK, Wilkinson JD. Candida onychomycosis. Evaluation of the role of candida species in nail disease. Br J Dermatol 1988; 118:47–58,

103. Haneke E. The nails in chronic mucocutaneous candidosis. 5th Annual Meeting of the Society for Cutaneous Ultrastructure Research, Nice, 20–21 May 1988, Book of Abstracts

104. Chugh KS, Sharma SC, Singh V, Sakhuja V, Jha V, Gupta KL. Spectrum of dermatological lesions in renal allograft recipient in a tropical environment. Dermatology 1994; 1988:108–12

105. Gülec AT, Demirbilcek M, Scskin D et al. Superficial fungal infection in 102 renal transplant recipients. A case control. J Am Acad Dermatol 2003; 49:187–92

106. Virgili A, Zampino MR, La Malfa V, Strumia R, Bedali PL. Prevalence of superficial dermatomycoses in 73 renal transplant recipients. Dermatology 1999; 1999:31–4

107. Weglowska J, Szepietowski J, Walow B, Szepietowski T. Onychomycosis in renal transplant recipient. Part II. Mycological aspects. Mikol Lek 2003; 10:307–11

108. Boonchai W, Kulthanan K, Maungprasat C, Suthipinithathan P. Clinical characteristics and mycology of onychomycosis in autoimmune patients. J Med Assoc Thai 2003; 86:995–1000

109. Tlacuilo-Parra A, Guevara-Gutierrez E, Mayorga J, Carcia de la Torre S, Salzar-Paramo M. Onychomycosis in systemic lupus erythematosus. A case control study. J Rheumatol 2003; 30:1491–4

110. Cribier B, Mena ML, Rey D et al. Nail changes in patients infected with human immunodeficiency virus. Arch Dermatol 2000; 134:1216–20

111. Dompmartin D, Domptmartin A, Deluol AM, Grosshans E, Coulaud JP. Onychomycoses and AIDS. Clinical and laboratory findings in 62 patients. Int J Dermatol 1990; 29:337–9

112. Rongioletti F, Persi A, Tripodi S, Rebora A. A proximal white subungual onychomycosis: a sign of immunodeficiency. J Am Acad Dermatol 1994; 30:129–30

113. Silva-Lizama E, Logemann N. Proximal white sub-ungual onychomycosis in AIDS. Int J Dermatol 1996; 35:290

114. Tosti A, Piraccini BM, Mariani R, Stinchi C, Buttasi C. Are local and systemic conditions important for the development of onychomycosis? Eur J Dermatol 1998; 8:41–4

115. Piérard GE. Onychomycosis and other superficial fungal infections on the foot in the elderly: a pan-European survey. Dermatology 2001; 202:220–4

Anatomy

The nail unit lies immediately above the periostium of the distal phalanx and consists of a keratinized product, the nail plate and four specialized epithelia: the proximal nail fold, the nail matrix, the nail bed and the hyponychium (Figure 2.1).[1,2]

Nail plate

The nail plate is a fully keratinized multilayered sheet of cornified cells. From the 15th week of embryonic life, nail plate production occurs continuously and thereafter almost uniformly throughout life.[1] The nail plate is almost rectangular in shape and translucent. It appears pink because of the blood vessels of the underlying nail bed. The nail plate adheres tightly to the nail bed, since the horny layer of the nail bed partially contributes to the formation of the ventral nail plate.[3] The nail plate has a somewhat loose attachment, along its lateral borders.[4]

Proximally and laterally, the nail plate is surrounded by the proximal and lateral folds, whereas its distal margin is free. Detachment of the nail plate from the underlying tissues occurs at the hyponychium, which marks the separation of the nail from the digit. The nail plate's free edge appears white due to the presence of air in the subungual space. This space frequently contains keratinous debris, especially in the toenails.

The proximal part of the fingernails, especially the thumbs, shows a whitish, opaque, half-moon-shaped area, the lunula, which is the visible portion of the nail matrix. The shape of the lunula determines the shape of the free edge of the nail plate.

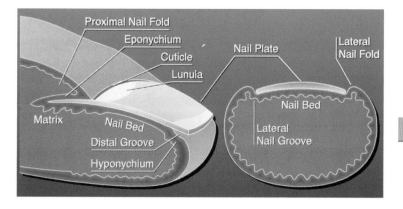

Figure 2.1

Sagittal and transverse section through finger nail.

More than 90% of fingernails show a thin distal transverse white band, the onychocorneal band, which marks the most distal portion of firm attachment of the nail plate to the nail bed.[5] This area represents an important anatomical barrier against environmental and microbial hazards.

In transverse sections, the nail plate consists of three portions: dorsal nail plate, intermediate nail plate and ventral nail plate.[6] The dorsal and intermediate portions of the nail plate are produced by the nail matrix and consist of hard keratins. The intermediate nail plate, which comes from the distal matrix, represents two-thirds of the whole nail thickness. The ventral portion of the nail plate is produced by the nail bed and is formed by soft keratins. The thickness of this portion of the nail plate considerably increases in nail bed disorders.

Nail matrix

The nail matrix consists of a proliferative epithelium that keratinizes in the absence of a granular layer. Maturation and differentiation of nail matrix keratinocytes lead to the formation of the superficial and intermediate layers of the nail plate. The site of nail matrix keratinization can be recognized in histological sections as an eosinophilic band (keratogenous zone). In this area, nail matrix keratinocytes show nuclear fragmentation and condensation of cytoplasm.

In longitudinal sections the matrix consists of a proximal (dorsal) and a distal (ventral) region. Proximal nail matrix keratinocytes give rise to the upper portion of the nail plate, whereas distal nail matrix keratinocytes produce its intermediate portion.

The nail matrix epithelium contains melanocytes. Although nail matrix melanocytes are usually quiescent, they may start to produce melanin in a large number of physiological and pathological conditions. This is more common in Black and Asian populations than in Caucasians. The nail growth rates range from 1.8 to 4.8 mm/month in fingernails and 1.3 to 1.8 mm/month in toenails. This gradually declines with age.[7] Complete replacement of a fingernail requires 4–6 months and that of a toenail 12–18 months. Linear nail growth may also increase in some physiological and pathological circumstances and may be influenced by drugs. The triazole derivatives itraconazole[8] and fluconazole[9] have been reported to enhance nail growth, although the mechanism has not been established. Terbinafine may also induce an increase of linear nail growth.[10]

Nail bed

The nail bed epithelium consists of several cell layers and extends from the lunula to the hyponychium. Nail bed keratinization occurs in the absence of a granular layer and gives rise to the ventral nail plate. This corresponds to about one-fifth of the terminal nail thickness and it can be recognized in histological sections because of its mild eosinophilia.

The nail bed dermoepidermal architecture shows a distinctive arrangement, with longitudinal grooves and ridges extending from the lunula to the hyponychium. The nail bed capillaries run longitudinally along these nail bed grooves.

The nail bed epithelium is so adherent to the nail plate that it remains attached to the under-surface of the nail when this is avulsed.

Hyponychium

The hyponychium is normally covered by the nail plate's free margin, but becomes visible in nail biters or when the nail plate is cut very short.

Its epithelium is similar to that of plantar or volar skin and it keratinizes through the formation of a granular layer. Cornified hyponychial cells accumulate in the subungual space, especially in toenails.

Proximal nail fold

The proximal nail plate is surrounded and partially covered by the proximal nail fold, which overlies about a quarter of the nail plate. Adhesion between the proximal nail fold and nail plate is tight due to the presence of the cuticle, which is firmly attached to the superficial nail plate. The cuticle, which is continuously formed by keratinization of the proximal nail fold, consists of a thin layer of orthokeratotic cells.

The proximal nail fold consists of a dorsal portion that is anatomically similar to the skin of the dorsum of the digit and a ventral portion that continues proximally with the proximal matrix.

References

1. Zaias N. The Nail in Health and Disease, 2nd edn. Norwalk, Appleton & Lange, 1990

2. Baran R, Dawber RPR. Diseases of the Nails and their Management (3rd edn). Oxford, Blackwell, 2001

3. Johnson M, Cosmaish JS, Shuster S. Nail is produced by the normal nail bed: a controversy resolved. Br J Dermatol 1991; 125:27–9

4. Baran R, De Doncker P. Lateral edge involvement indicates poor prognosis for treating onychomycosis with the new systemic antifungals. Acta Derm Venereol 1996; 73:82–3

5. Sonnex TS, Griffiths WAD, Nicol WJ. The nature and significance of the transverse white band of human nails. Semin Dermatol 1981; 10:12–16

6. Forslind B. Biophysical studies of the normal nail. Acta Derm Venereol 1970; 50:161–8

7. Bean WB. Nail growth. Twenty-five year's observation. Arch Intern Med 1968; 122:359–61

8. De Doncker P, Pierard G. Acquired nail beading in patients receiving itraconazole. An indicator of faster nail growth? A study using optical profilometry. Clin Exp Dermatol 1994; 19:404–6

9. Shelley WB, Shelley ED. Portrait of a practice. Cutis 1992; 49:386

10. Faergemann J, Anderson C, Hersle K et al. Double-blind, parallel-group comparison of terbinafine and griseofulvin in the treatment of toenail onychomycosis. J Am Acad Dermatol 1995; 32:750–3

Clinical patterns correlated with routes of entry

A fungus gains entry to the nail by four main routes, each resulting in different clinical patterns of infection.[1,2] These are described below.

Via the distal subungual area and the lateral nail groove (Figure 3.1)

This leads to distal lateral subungual onychomycosis (DLSO) (Figure 3.2a–i). The fungus invades the horny layer of the hyponychium and/or the nail bed, then the under-surface of the nail plate, which becomes opaque. This causes thickening of the horny layer, raising the free edge of the nail plate with disruption of the normal nail plate–nail

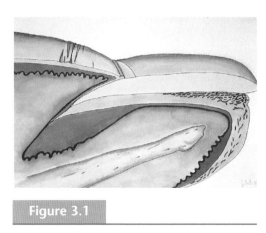

Figure 3.1

Distal lateral subungual onychomycosis (DSLO).

bed attachment. The disease spreads proximally against the stream of nail growth. Sometimes a yellow brown discoloration is observed. *Trichophyton rubrum* is the most common fungal invader, *T. mentagrophytes* var. *interdigitale* is much less common and *Epidermophyton floccosum* is rare. In contrast to this form, DLSO may also appear as primary onycholysis with a minimum of hyperkeratosis, especially in fingernails (Figure 3.3a,b). Primary onycholysis may be associated with the presence of *Candida* (Figure 3.4a,b). Overriding of the toes and repeated microtrauma of the nail against the shoes may create an area of onycholysis favourable to the invasion of microorganisms. In such cases, mixed infection due to *T. rubrum* and *Pseudomonas* is not exceptional (Figure 3.5). The clinical significance of nail invasion or colonization by fungi which are not normally pathogenic needs to be carefully considered in the light of laboratory findings. The nail bed infection in DLSO caused by *T. rubrum* is the result of the fungus spreading from the plantar (Figure 3.6)[3] and palmar surface of the feet and hands, a pattern seen in the one-hand-two-foot tinea syndrome (Figure 3.7a,b). The involved palm has reduced sweating and feels dry.[4] The omnipresent sign of the chronic dermatophytosis syndrome[5] is tinea pedis of the soles. The starting signs of the lifelong syndrome are minute plantar vesicles of 1 mm diameter and collarettes

3

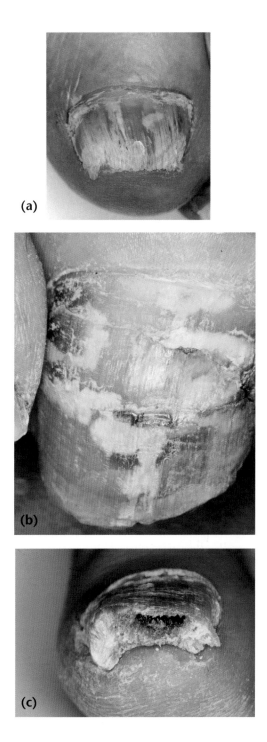

(a)

(b)

(c)

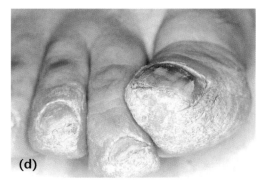

(d)

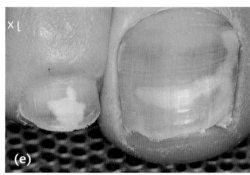

(e)

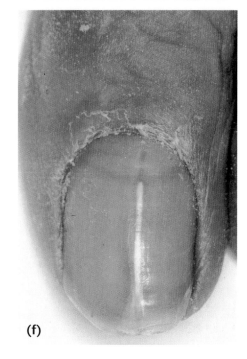

(f)

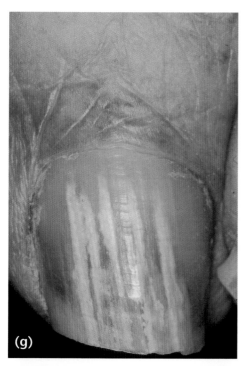

(g)

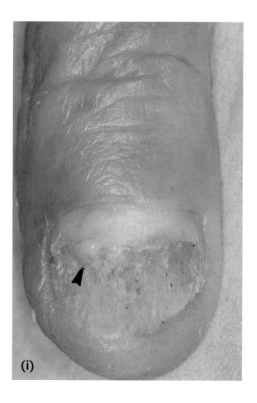

(i)

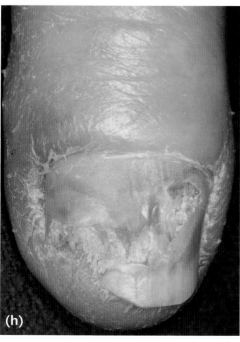

(h)

Figure 3.2

(a) DLSO due to *T. rubrum*. (b) DLSO associated with various colours. (c) DLSO associated with hyperkeratosis and onycholysis. (d) Chronic dermatophytic disease due to *T. rubrum*. (e) Association of DLSO and superficial white onychomychysis (SWO) due to *T. interdigitale*. (f) DLSO distal to proximal single streak. (g) DLSO distal to proximal multiple streaks. (h) DLSO due to *Aspergillus*. (i) Same patient presenting with an abscess of the exposed nail bed.

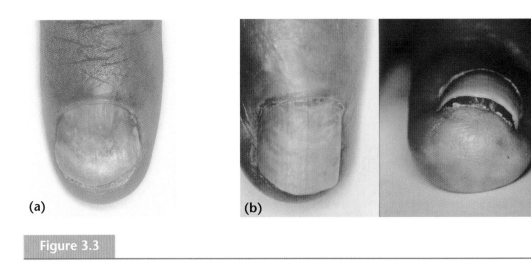

(a) DLSO with onycholysis due to *T. rubrum*. (b) DLSO with onycholysis associated with *Mucor*.

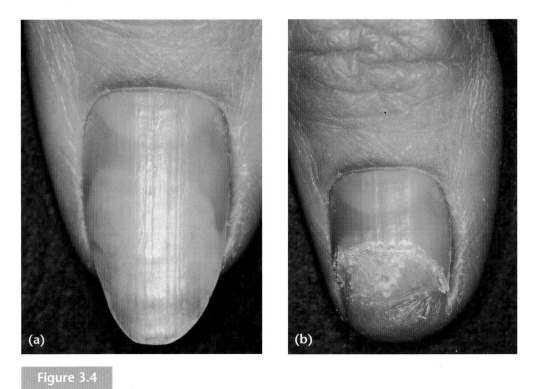

(a) *Candida* onycholysis. (b) Same patient after nail debridement.

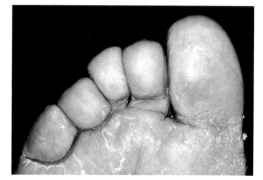

Figure 3.6

Tinea pedis.

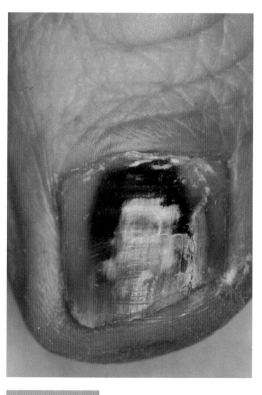

Figure 3.5

Mixed infection due to *T. rubrum* and *Pseudomonas*.

that are the site of abundant hyphae. The vesicles dry and lose their old vesicle tops, leaving a keratinous collarette. These lesions involve only the thick skin of the soles. After the initial infection of the soles, other sites of the host become infected, especially the nail bed, leading to DLSO with hyperkeratosis, its principal sign.[5] Clinically severe *T. rubrum* plantar infections that manifest as the 'moccasin-type' are found in less than 10% of patients.

T. mentagrophytes var. *interdigitale* (TI) produces a chronic syndrome[6] character-

ized by, on the one hand, the episodic occurrence of groups of pruritic multilocular vesicles, or bullae. These are larger than 2 mm and can be found in the thin skin of the plantar arch and along the sides of the foot and heel adjacent to the thick plantar stratum corneum and, on the other hand, by superficial white onychomycosis. These bullae or vesicles, which appear during periods of stress, such as wearing occlusive shoes, are frequently the first evidence of an ongoing *T. mentagrophytes* var. *interdigitale* infection noticed by the patient. This periplantar distribution usually differs from that produced by *T. rubrum* involving the thick plantar stratum corneum of the sole of the foot, as seen above.

The lesions produced in the toe spaces by *T. interdigitale* are more often vesicular and pruritic than those produced by *T. rubrum* but may affect the dorsal skin of the toe around the nail and the occluded sides of the toe.[7] Black fungi such as *T. rubrum nigricans* may present as longitudinal melanonychia (see Figures 4.23 and 4.24).

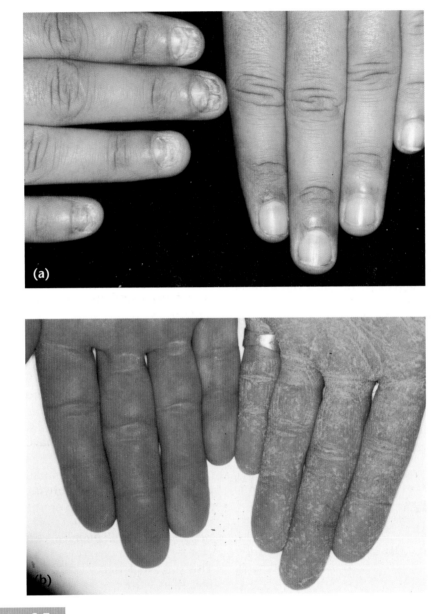

Figure 3.7

(a) One hand/two-foot syndrome with fingernails also affected. (b) Ventral aspect of a similar patient.

Organisms such as *Scytalidium dimidia-tum* which mimic the pattern of disease caused by dermatophytes (chronic pseudo dermatophytic syndrome) produce the clinical pattern of DLSO, but this is often associated with onycholysis, and sometimes paronychia, especially in fingernails (Figure 3.8).

Via the dorsal surface of the nail plate (Figure 3.9), producing superficial onychomycosis (Figure 3.10a–c)

Superficial white onychomycosis (SWO) is normally confined to the toenails. The causative organisms produce the clinical picture of small, white patches with distinct edges on the dorsal nail plate. These latter coalesce and may gradually cover the whole nail. The chalky white surface becomes roughened and the texture softer than normal. *T. mentagrophytes var. inter-digitale* is responsible for more than 90% of the cases. *T. rubrum* is rarely encountered in immunocompetent patients.[7] Superficial scraping gets rid of the white patches.

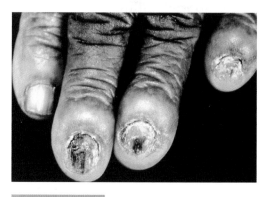

Figure 3.8

DLSO due to *Scytalidium dimidatum* with associated paronychia.

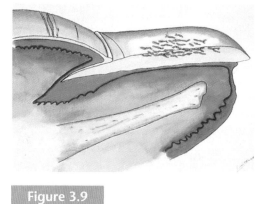

Figure 3.9

Superficial onychomycosis.

Lesions of SWO may range from minimal to extensive and are part of a syndrome caused by *T. interdigitale* that includes interdigital tinea pedis and vesicular arch-type tinea pedis. Superficial infections caused by non-dermatophyte moulds such as *Aspergillus terreus*, *Fusarium oxysporum* or *Acremonium* spp. are more often seen in patients in tropical and subtropical environments (Table 3.1). Children presenting with SWO may have *Candida albicans* infection.

Superficial black onychomycosis (SBO), the counterpart of SWO, is very rare. Cases reported have been produced by *T. rubrum* and *Scytalidium dimidiatum*.[7,8]

The proximal nail fold may be mildly inflamed,[9] the nail is diffusely opaque and friable with a pigmentation varying from homogeneous white to patchy yellow-brown.

Besides the classic clinical pattern of superficial nail invasion, two other sub-types have been recorded:[10] (1) SWO with deep penetration;[9,10] (2) dual invasion of

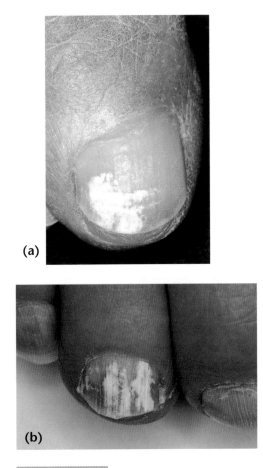

(a)

(b)

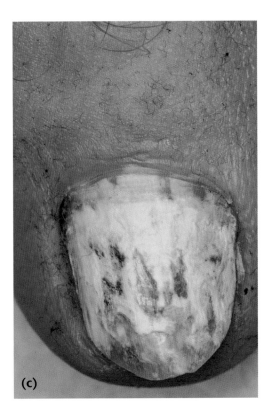

(c)

Figure 3.10

(a) SWO. (b) Association of SWO with proximal white subungual onychomycosis (PWSO) (bipolar type). (c) Deep penetration from SWO.

the nail plate, superficial and ventral. The clues to deep invasion of the nail plate are twofold: an inability to clear the discoloration by scraping the nail and SWO starting from beneath the proximal nail fold due to fungal infection of the ventral aspect of its eponychial segment. The bipolar type is encountered in young children (with thin nails)[11] and very

often in HIV-positive subjects,[12] where it is sometimes difficult to guess if the origin of the infection is due to superficial involvement or to proximal white subungual onychomychosis.

This new subdivision of SWO reflects previously unrecognized variants with therapeutic implications. Topical anti-

TABLE 3.1	Fungi isolated in superficial onychomycosis		
DERMATOPHYTES	**YEASTS**	**MOULDS**	
T. mentagrophytes interdigitale *T. rubrum* *Microsporum canis* *Microsporum persicolor*	*Candida albicans*	*Aspergillus* spp. *Fusarium* spp. *Acremonium* spp. **Pseudo dermatophytes** *Onychocola canadensis* *Scytalidium dimidiatum*	

fungal agents will be used when the disease is restricted to the dorsum of the nail. Systemic drugs either in isolation or – better – in combination with topical treatment are mandatory when deep penetration or ventral fungal infection are observed with histological confirmation.

Combined distal and lateral subungual and white superficial onychomycosis in the toenails (Figure 3.11)

In the Gupta and Summerbell series,[13] 39 (0.9%) of 4411 patients had the combination DLSO and SWO, compared with 417 (9.4%) and 111 (2.5%) who had DLSO or SWO, respectively. After controlling for age and sex in the general population, the projected prevalence rates of DLSO, SWO, and combined DLSO and SWO in the province of Ontario, Canada were 7.1%, 1.5% and 5%, respectively. The combination of DLSO and SWO in the toenails of an individual occurred more frequently than that predicted by chance. Nine (0.2%) of 4411 subjects had DLSO and SWO on the same nail. In 23 (59%) of 39 subjects both the DLSO and SWO were associated with *Trichophyton menta-*

grophytes. In the remaining 16 subjects other organisms cultured were *T. rubrum*, *Acremonium* spp., *Aspergillus* spp., *Fusarium oxysporum* and *Onychocola canadensis*. In 33 (84.6%) of 39 subjects

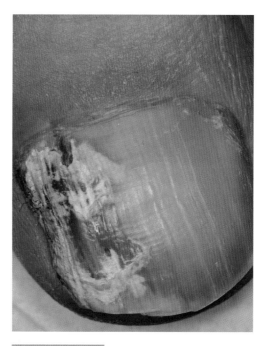

Figure 3.11

Combined DLSO and SWO on the same toenail.

with the combination of DLSO and SWO on the toenails, the same fungal organism was associated with both the DLSO and SWO. It may also occur where a toenail is occluded by an overlying malformed adjacent toe.

In conclusion, when both DLSO and SWO are concurrently present in the toenails of an individual, partitioned sampling (i.e. sampling for each of the two types of onychomycosis) may provide a better understanding of the different organisms associated with the onychomycosis and the relationship between the two types of onychomycosis.

T. rubrum demonstrating three different entry sites is an unusual finding.[14]

Via the under-surface of the proximal nail fold (Figures 3.12 and 3.13a–c)

Among the major patterns of fungal nail plate invasion, proximal white subungual onychomycosis (PWSO) is a specific form where infection first appears from below the proximal nail fold and spreads distally under the nail plate (Figure 3.13a). It may affect the finger as well as the toenails. The stratum corneum on the ventral aspect of the proximal nail fold appears to be the primary site of fungal invasion, but when the fungus reaches the matrix, it mainly spreads to the lower part of the nail plate. The main clinical feature, a white patch, visible through the transparent and smooth nail plate, appears from beneath the normal cuticle and then extends distally. The ventral aspect of the proximal nail fold may show a microscopic focus

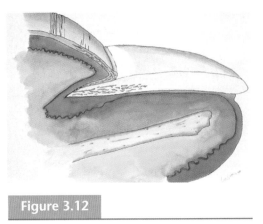

Figure 3.12

Proximal white subungual onychomycosis (PWSO).

of acute epidermal and dermal involvement whose histopathological appearances were described by Zaias in 1990.[15]

However, could PWSO be a complication of systemic spread?[16] Recently, the question of a potential role[17] of lymphatic or deep spread in some types of onychomycosis has been raised. In this proposal fungal infection or auto-infection might originate from a deeper site rather than a new external infection. In such cases, it was suggested that the appearance of PWSO might represent reactivation that would follow initial spread and sequestration, for example, in lymph nodes,[18] with subsequent systemic dissemination either through retrograde lymphatic[19] or haematogenous spread into the nail matrix and nail bed. The dermatophyte antigenaemia seen in patients with foot infections would be in keeping with such a mechanism.

In addition to the clinical picture described above, PSWO may present in a variety of other forms. There may be

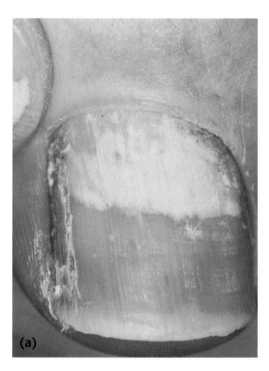

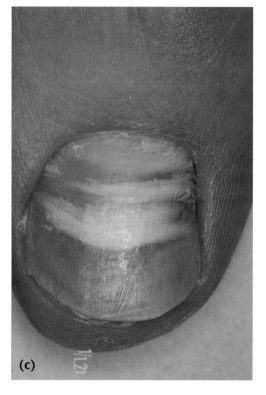

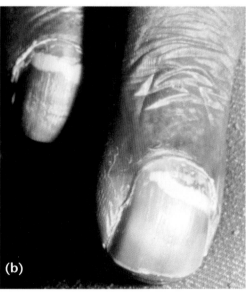

Figure 3.13

(a) PWSO. (b) PWSO presenting as a transverse leuconychia (with a single band). (c) PWSO presenting as a transverse leuconychia (with a multiple band).

proximal to distal longitudinal leucony-chia affecting a single digit, an isolated transverse leuconychial band (Figure 3.13b), or there may be multiple trans-verse bands separated by areas of nail, which are both clinically and histologi-cally normal, affecting the same digit (Figure 3.13c). Finally there is a rapidly developing form of PWSO recorded in patients suffering from HIV infection. The fungal infection, more frequent when the CD4+ cell count is less than 450 cells/mm[3],[20] may spread to all the fingers (even over the paronychium[21]) and toenails. This is caused by pre-existing tinea pedis due to *T. rubrum* that pre-dates immunosuppression.

PWSO is usually caused by *T. rubrum*. Exceptionally, *T. megninii*, *T. schoenleinii* or *Epidermophyton floccosum* have been reported. Recently proximal subungual onychomycosis without paronychia due to *Candida* has been demonstrated in chronic mucocutaneous candidosis.[22]

Sometimes, PWSO due to *T. rubrum* may extend to the superficial nail plate, producing a clinical picture that resem-bles SWO. This is usually seen in finger-nails, but has also been described in children who have thin toenails[11] and in HIV-positive subjects.[23]

Proximal subungual onychomycosis secondary to paronychia (Figure 3.14)

Paronychia is observed mainly in adult women (housework) and affects partic-ularly the index, middle finger and thumb of the dominant hand.[24] Frequent manual work with carbohydrate-containing foods and moisture, macer-ation, occlusion (latex), hyperhidrosis and acrocyanosis favour the disease. The first step in the development of chronic paronychia is mechanical infection or chemical trauma that produces cuticle damage. At that time the epidermal bar-rier of the ventral aspect of the proximal nail fold is destroyed and the area is sud-denly exposed to a variety of environ-mental hazards. Irritants and allergens with immediate hypersensitivity (type I)

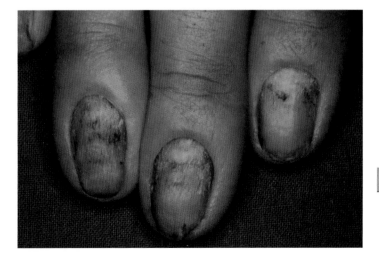

Figure 3.14

PWSO with paronychia. (Image courtesy of B. Schubert, France.)

reaction to food ingredients may then produce an inflammation of the nail fold and nail matrix, which interferes with the normal nail growth. Usually the nail fold inflammatory reaction affects the lateral portion of the matrix leading to nail plate deformity on the same side, appearing as irregular transverse ridging or a dark narrow strip down one or both lateral borders of the nail.

The thickened free end of the erythematous proximal nail fold becomes rounded, retracted and loses the ability to form a cuticle. The disease tends to run a protracted course interrupted by subacute exacerbations due to secondary *Candida* spp.[24] and bacterial infection with formation of a small abscess in the space formed between the proximal nail fold and the nail plate. Diabetes mellitus and other hormonal disturbances and drugs such as corticosteroids, cytotoxic agents and antibiotics may exacerbate *Candida* paronychia.

Depending on the major etiological factors involved, chronic paronychia can be classified into the following types:[25]

1. Contact allergy (topical drug ingredients, rubber, etc.).
2. Food contact hypersensitivity.
3. *Candida* hypersensitivity (a similar reaction to that suggested in some patients with recurrent vaginitis).
4. Irritant reaction (irritant chronic paronychia may subsequently acquire a secondary hypersensitivity and develop chronic food hypersensitivity paronychia and/or *Candida* hypersensitivity paronychia).
5. *Candida* paronychia.

True *Candida* paronychia is uncommon in temperate climates except in patients with chronic mucocutaneous candidosis and HIV infection. In this condition proximal nail fold inflammation is usually associated with proximal onycholysis or onychomycosis due to *Candida*, which can be isolated both from the proximal nail fold and clipping of the affected nail plate.

In contrast to *Candida* infection, non-dermatophyte moulds such as *Fusarium* (Figure 3.15) may produce subacute paronychia accompanied by proximal white onychomycosis, especially in immunocompromised individuals.[26] *Scopulariopsis brevicaulis* (Figure 3.16) may be responsible for identical features with a white or yellow discoloration of the nail plate.[27] Proximal subungual onychomycosis may also be associated with marked periungual inflammation and black discoloration of the lunula region due to *Aspergillus niger*.[28]

6. Bacterial paronychia.

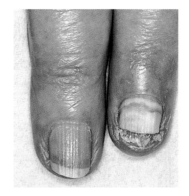

Figure 3.15

PWSO due to *Fusarium*.

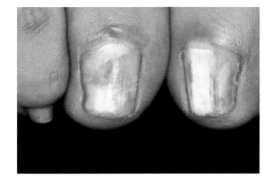

Figure 3.16

PWSO with paronychia due to *Scopulariopsis brevicaulis*.

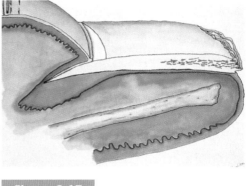

Figure 3.17

Endonyx onychomycosis.

The existence of chronic paronychia solely attributable to bacteria is debatable, although in some patients the only readily identifiable aetiological agents are bacteria, usually Gram-negative forms.
7. Systemic drugs.
8. Tumours involving the paronychial area.

Endonyx onychomycosis (Figure 3.17)

A new form of invasion of the nail plate by fungal elements has been described.[29,30] The dermatophyte reaches the nail plate via the pulp as in the DLSO type. Instead of infecting the nail bed however, the fungus penetrates the distal nail keratin where it forms milky white patches without subungual hyperkeratosis or onycholysis. Endonyx infection has been described with *T. soudanense* (Figure 3.18), but may also be due to *T. violaceum* infection. Both dermatophytes cause endothrix hair shaft invasion in tinea capitis.

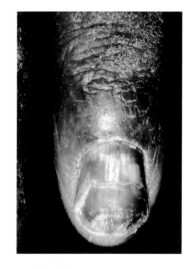

Figure 3.18

Endonyx onychomycosis due to *Trichophyton soudanense*.

Total dystrophic onychomycosis (TDO) (Figure 3.19)

Secondary TDO (Figure 3.20) represents the most advanced form of all the types

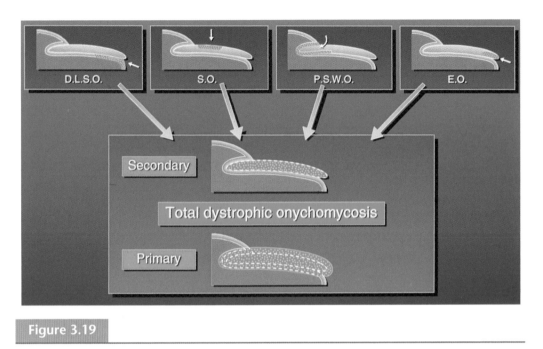

Figure 3.19

Development of total dystrophic onychomycosis.

described above. The nail crumbles and disappears, leaving a thickened, abnormal nail bed retaining keratotic nail debris.

In the new form of total nail dystrophy observed in patients with AIDS, infection appears to have spread from under the proximal nail fold (PWSO) but this has not been established in all cases. The dorsum of the nail plate may also be involved. The term acute TDO might be appropriate for this type of infection.

In contrast to secondary TDO, primary TDO is observed only in patients suffering from chronic mucocutaneous candidosis (CMCC) (Figure 3.21) or in other

immunodeficiency states[31] (Table 3.2). *Candida* invasion rapidly involves all the tissues of the nail apparatus. The thickening of the soft tissues results in a swollen distal phalanx that is more bulbous than clubbed. The nail plate is thickened, opaque and yellow-brown in colour. Hyperkeratotic areas secondary to *Candida* invasion may develop in skin adjacent to the nail. Oral candidosis is generally present in these patients. This syndrome, which usually presents in childhood or infancy, recurs despite treatment. Dual or sole infection with dermatophytes may occur in patients with CMCC. Isolated nail candidosis has also been associated with genetically determined ICAM-I deficiency.[32]

TABLE 3.2	Subtypes of chronic mucocutaneous candidosis (CMCC)*		
TYPE†		**PATTERN OF INHERITANCE**	**SPECIAL CLINICAL/ IMMUNOLOGICAL FEATURES**
CMCC			
Without endocrinopathy (212050)		Recessive	Childhood onset
With endocrinopathy‡ (240300)		Recessive	Chilhood onset. Patients have the polyendocrinopathy syndrome
Without endocrinopathy (114580)		Dominant	Childhood onset
With endocrinopathy		Dominant	Childhood onset. Associated with hypothyroidism
Sporadic CMCC		None known	Childhood onset
CMCC with keratitis		None known	Childhood onset. Associated with keratitis
Late-onset CMCC§		None known	Onset in adult life. Associated with thymoma

Reproduced from ref. 31, with permission.

* While originally severe CMCC (e.g. *candida* granuloma) was described in association with specific subtypes it is now apparent that extensive infection, including hyperkeratotic candidosis and dermatophytosis, is not specific to any one variety.

† Numbers in parentheses are McKusick numbers.

‡ The main endocrine diseases seen with this variety are hypoparathyroidism and hypoadrenalism.

§ Other late-onset types have been recorded, e.g. with systemic lupus erythematosus, but as they are usually associated with systemic corticosteroid therapy, they have been excluded as secondary candidosis.

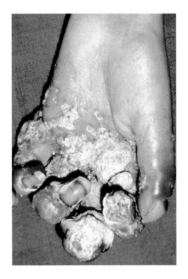

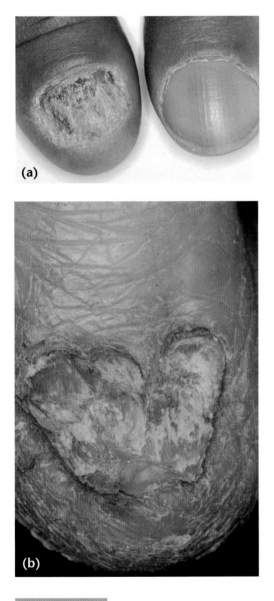

(a)

(b)

Figure 3.21

Primary total dystrophic onychomycosis.
(Image courtesy of D. Leroy, Caen.)

Figure 3.20

(a,b) Secondary total dystrophic
onychomycosis.

References

1. Zaias N. Onychomycosis. Arch Dermatol 1972; 105:263–74

2. Baran R, Hay RJ, Tosti A, Haneke E. A new classification of onychomycosis. Br J Dermatol 1998; 119:567–71

3. Evans EGV. Causative pathogens in onychomycosis and the possibility of treatment resistance: a review. J Am Acad Dermatol 1998; 38:S32–S36

4. Daniel CR III, Gupta AK, Daniel MP, Daniel CM. Two feet-one hand syndrome: a retrospective multicenter survey. Int J Dermatol 1997; 36:658–60

5. Zaias N, Rebell G. Chronic dermatophytosis syndrome due to *Trichophyton rubrum*. Int J Dermatol 1996; 35:614–17

6. Zaias N, Rebell G. Clinical and mycological status of the *Trichophyton mentagrophytes* (*interdigitale*) syndrome of chronic dermatophytosis of the skin and nails. Int J Dermatol 2003; 42:779–88

7. Badillet G. Mélanonychies superficielles. Bull Soc Fr Mycol Med 1988; 17:335–40

8. Meisel CW, Quadripur SA. Onychomycosis due to *Hendersonula toruloidea*. Hautnah Myk 1992; 6:232–4

9. Piraccini BM, Tosti A. White superficial onychomycosis. Arch Dermatol 2004; 140:696–701

10. Baran R, Hay R, Perrin C. Superficial white onychomycosis revisited. J Eur Acad Dermatol Venereol 2004; 18:569–71

11. Ploysangan T, Lucky AW. Childhood white superficial onychomycosis caused by *Trichophyton rubrum*. J Am Acad Dermatol 1997; 36:29–32

12. Ravnborg L, Baastrup N, Svejgaard E. Onychomycosis in HIV-infected patients. Acta Derm Venereol 1997; 78:151–2

13. Gupta AK, Summerbel R. Combined distal and lateral subungual and white superficial onychomycosis in the toenails. J Am Acad Dermatol 1999; 6:938–44

14. Baran R, Haneke E, Tosti A. *Trichophyton rubrum* demonstrating three different entry sites. Mikologia Lekarska 1958; 5:47

15. Zaias N. The Nail in Health and Disease, 2nd edn. Norwalk, CT, Appleton & Lange, 1990

16. Baran R, McCloone N, Hay RJ. Could proximal white onychomycosis (PWSO) be a complication of systemic spread? The lessons to be learned from Maladie dermatophytique and other deep infections. Br J Dermatol 2005; 153:1023–5

17. Hay RJ, Baran R. Deep dermatophytosis: rare infections or common, but unrecognised complications of lymphatic spread? Curr Opin Infect Dis 2004; 17:77–9

18. Arievitch AM, Shetziruli LT. I Nail Pathology. Tbilisi, Metzniereba, 1976:76–100

19. Pagliaro JA, White SI. Specific skin lesions occurring in a patient with Hodgkin's lymphoma. Australas J Dermatol 1999; 40:41–3

20. Daniel CR III, Norton LA, Scher RK. The spectrum of nail disease in patients with immunodeficiency virus infection. J Am Acad Dermatol 1992; 27:93–7

21. Kaplan MH, Sadick N, McNutt S et al. Dermatologic findings and manifestations of AIDS. J Am Acad Dermatol 1987; 16:485–506

22. Baran R. Proximal subungual *Candida* onychomycosis. An unusual manifestation of chronic muco cutaneous candidosis. Br J Dermatol 1997; 137:286–8

23. Noppakun N, Head ES. Proximal white subungual onychomycosis in a patient with acquired immune deficiency syndrome. Int J Dermatol 1986; 25:586–7

24. Daniel CR, Daniel MP, Daniel CM, Sullivan S, Ellis G. Chronic paronychia and onycholysis. A thirteen-year experience. Cutis 1996, 58:397–401

25. Tosti A, Piraccini BM. Paronychia. In Amin S, Maibach HI, eds. Contact Urticaria Syndrome. Boca Raton, FL, CRC Press, 1997: 267–78

26. Baran R, Tosti A, Piraccini BM. Uncommon clinical patterns of *Fusarium* nail infection: report of three cases. Br J Dermatol 1997; 136:424–7

27. Tosti A, Piraccini BM, Strinchi C et al. Onychomycosis due to *Scopulariopsis brevicaulis:* clinical features and response to systemic antifungals. Br J Dermatol 1996; 135:799–802

28. Tosti A, Piraccini BM. Proximal subungual onychomycosis due to *Aspergillus niger*. Report of two cases. Br J Dermatol 1998; 139:152–69

29. Tosti A, Baran R, Piraccini BM, Fanti PA. "Endonyx" onychomycosis: a new modality of nail invasion by dermatophytic fungi. Acta Derm Venereol 1999; 79:52–3

30. Fletcher CL, Moore K, Hay RJ. Endonyx onychomycosis due to *T. soudanense* in two Somali siblings. Br J Dermatol 2001; 145:684–8

31. Coleman R, Hay RJ. Chronic mucocutaneous candidosis associated with hypothyroidism: a distinct syndrome? Br J Dermatol 1997; 136:24–9

32. Mangino M, Salpietro DC, Zuccarello D et al. A gene for familial isolated chronic nail candidiasis maps to chromosome 11p12–q12.1. Eur J Hum Genet 2003; 11:433–6.

Clinical differential diagnosis

Onychomycosis is so frequently encountered in daily practice that any nail dystrophy, especially one occurring in isolation, may be wrongly diagnosed. In addition, some entirely different dermatoses may cause similar nail alterations. This is due to the fact that the nail apparatus has a limited repertoire of reaction patterns and the nail plate covers and hides the very structures involved in the pathological process. Some examples are given below:[1-3]

Distal lateral subungual onychomycosis with prominent subungual hyperkeratosis

This can be mimicked by several inflammatory nail conditions, characterized by their protracted and recalcitrant courses.

1. **Psoriasis** (Figure 4.1) is the skin disease that most often produces nail changes and can mimic onychomycosis even histologically (see p. 57), especially in the HIV-positive patient.

    Subungual keratosis can be isolated or associated with onycholysis, leuconychia and distal splinter haemorrhages. As distortion and dystrophy of the nail plate may be seen in both onychomycosis and psoriasis, it may be impossible to diagnose psoriasis restricted to the nails on clinical grounds alone unless there is extensive pitting and/or the oil drop sign.

    Psoriatic nails are said to be more susceptible to fungal infection. Hence dual infection is not exceptional in toenails.

2. Skin changes and nail features in **Reiter's syndrome** may be indistinguishable from those of patients with psoriasis. However, a brownish-red hue of the nail bed lesions may suggest this condition.

3. **Repeated microtrauma.** Epithelial hyperplasia of the subungual tissues may result from repeated trauma.

4. **Pityriasis rubra pilaris** (Figure 4.2). In adult acute-onset type I pityriasis rubra pilaris nail involvement usually presents as distal subungual hyperkeratosis with moderate thickening of the nail bed, splinter haemorrhages and longitudinal ridging.

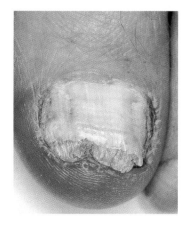

Figure 4.1

Psoriasis.

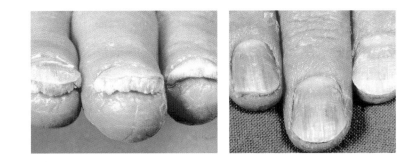

Figure 4.2

Pityriasis rubra pilaris.

5. **Norwegian (crusted) scabies** (Figure 4.3). The hyperkeratotic lesions are accompanied by large, psoriasis-like accumulations of scales under the nails and may resemble onychomycosis due to *Trichophyton rubrum* (cf. Figure 3.2c). The mites survive in these dystrophic nails and later colonize the skin, first around the nail plates; from there, they extend proximally. This type of scabies is most often seen in the old and infirm, the mentally ill and AIDS patients and during immunosuppression.

6. **Keratosis cristarum** (Figure 4.4) presents with a keratinizing process limited to the peripheral area of the

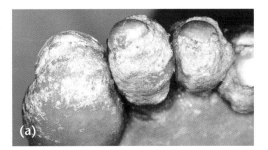

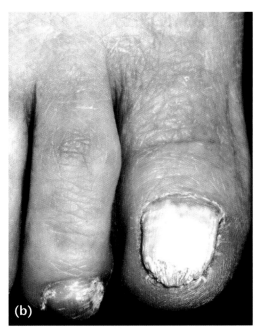

Figure 4.3

(a) Norwegian scabies. (b) Norwegian scabies mainly restricted to the great toenail (Coll G. Cremer.)

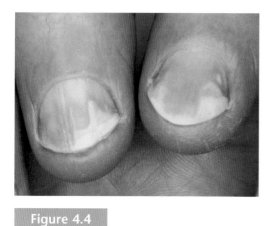

Figure 4.4

Keratosis cristarum.

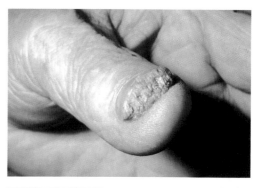

Figure 4.6

Lichen planus.

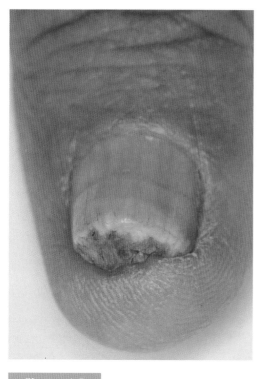

Figure 4.5

Darier's disease.

nail bed. It starts at the distal portion but may progress somewhat proximally. *Scopulariopsis brevicaulis* onychomycosis may present with identical changes.

7. **Darier's disease** (Figure 4.5). In typical cases the nails have longitudinal subungual pink or white streaks or both, and distal wedge-shaped subungual keratoses.

8. **Lichen planus** (Figure 4.6). Usually there is a progressive thinning and fluting of the nail and marked subungual hyperkeratosis may lift the nail plate. It may therefore be associated with onycholysis which can sometimes be seen in isolation.

9. **Chronic contact dermatitis** (Figure 4.7). The cause of nail changes is obvious when the eczema has a periungual distribution. It may be difficult to recognize in atopic dermatitis, discoid eczema, etc. The modifications of the nail result from disturbances of the matrix. These may present as thickening,

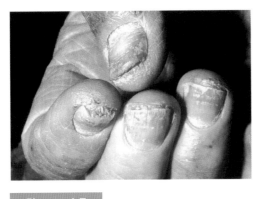

Figure 4.7

Chronic dermatitis.

pitting and transverse ridging sometimes leading to shedding of the nail. Exudative skin disease may occur with any chronic condition involving this area.

10. **Erythroderma** (Figure 4.8). In chronic erythroderma due to Sézary's syndrome, for example, nail changes are similar to those found in patients with type I pityriasis rubra pilaris.

11. **Pachyonychia congenita** (Figure 4.9). This is a hereditary ectodermal dysplasia with thickening of the nails which become yellow-brown tubular, hard and barrel-shaped. They project upward at their free edge while the subungual tissue is filled with keratotic material. The nail dystrophy usually appears within the first 6 months of life but later occurrence has been reported. Paronychia and onycholysis are common as well as recurrent shedding of the nail. Secondary *Candida* infection may occur.

12. **Acrokeratosis paraneoplastica** (Figure 4.10). This occurs in association with malignancy of the upper respiratory or digestive tract. In severe forms, the free edge is raised by subungual hyperkeratosis. The lesions resemble advanced psoriatic nail dystrophy and may progress to complete loss of the diseased nails.

13. **Bowen's disease** (Figure 4.11). Classic patterns in periungual involvement include hyperkeratotic or papillomatous and even warty proliferation; erosions; scaling of the nail fold; whitish cuticle; periungual swelling from deep tumour proliferation; ulceration of the lateral nail groove is sometimes crusted with granulation-like tissue beneath the scab.

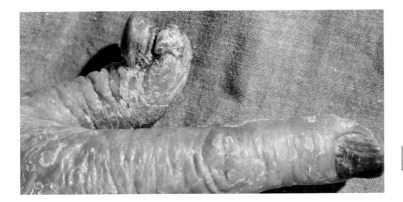

Figure 4.8

Sézary syndrome.

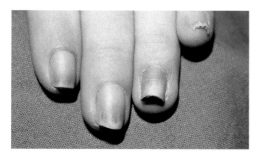

Figure 4.9

Familial pachyonychia congenita.
(Image courtesy of G. Moulin, Lyon.)

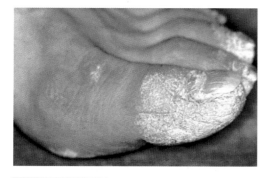

Figure 4.10

Acrokeratosis paraneoplastica.

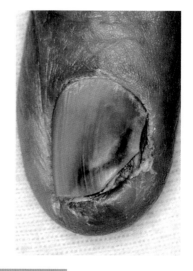

Figure 4.11

Bowen's disease.

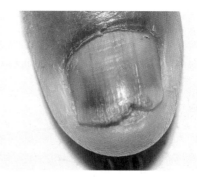

Figure 4.12

Lichen planus onycholysis. (Image
courtesy of S. Goettmann-Bonvallot, Paris).

Distal lateral subungual onychomycosis with marked onycholysis

Onycholysis can appear in many different conditions (Figures 4.12–4.14, Table 4.1).

In fingernails, primary onycholysis is more frequently associated with secondary invasion by *Candida* and/or *Pseudomonas*. It should be differentiated from nail plate–nail bed separation due to overzealous cleaning with an orange stick, for example.

Traumatic onycholysis of the toenails may present differently to that of fingernails. The diagnosis is obvious when the nail plate–nail bed separation appears after strenuous exercise in new footwear.

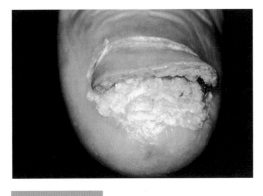

Figure 4.13

Psoriasis.

Occasionally, a blackish hue may be the only presentation and is often due to the second toe overriding the big toe, which results in lateral subungual triangular haemorrhage (Figure 4.14). This is more common in women for obvious reasons. Patients with the various forms of epidermolysis bullosa are more susceptible to onycholysis. In Bowen's disease onycholysis is often associated with oozing erosion.

Superficial white onychomycosis

Superficial friability can be produced by keratin granulations due to nail varnish or to base coat (Figure 4.15).

The parakeratotic psoriatic cells, which usually disappear from the nail surface, leaving pitting, may be abnormally adherent to each other for a long period (Figure 4.16), producing white superficial patches. An identical presentation may be observed in alopecia areata.

Proximal subungual white onychomycosis without paronychia

This type of fungal infection, which may present with varied features, can be mimicked by:

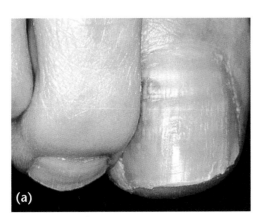

(a)

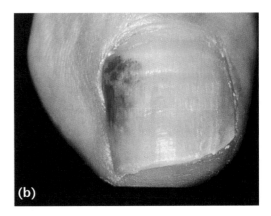

(b)

Figure 4.14

(a) Repeated minor trauma due to overriding of the second toe. (b) Subungual haematoma in the same patient.

TABLE 4.1	Differential diagnosis of fungal onycholysis

Nail infection
    Bacterial: *Pseudomonas, Proteus mirabilis*
    Viral: herpes simplex, warts

Dermatological disease
    Bullous diseases
    Contact dermatitis, atopic dermatitis
    Cutaneous T lymphoma
    Langerhans histiocytosis
    Lichen planus (Figure 4.12)
    Pachyonychia congenita
    Psoriasis/Reiter's syndrome (Figure 4.13)
    Subungual tumours (benign or malignant)

Chemical causes
    Alkalis, mineral oils
    Cosmetics (depilatories)
    Detergents and solvents
    Fluorhydric acid
    Sodium hypochlorite
    Sugar

Physical causes
    Burn
    Foreign body implantation
    Manicure
    Occupational factors
    Overlapping of the toes
    Repeated microtrauma (Figure 4.14)
    Sport enthusiasts

Systemic conditions
    Acrokeratosis paraneoplastica
    Cancers
    Iron deficiency
    Lupus erythematosus, scleroderma
    Pregnancy
    Raynaud's disease
    Thyroidism
    Yellow nail syndrome

Congenital and/or hereditary disease
    Epidermolysis bullosa
    Hereditary partial onycholysis (Schulze)

Drugs
    Cytotoxics (bleomycin, 5-fluorouracil, docetaxel, placitaxel, etc.)
    Etretinate, acitretin, isotretinoin
    Psoralens, cyclines, fluoroquinolones (responsible for photo-onycholysis)

- Congenital transverse leuconychia (Figure 4.17).
- Longitudinal leuconychia in Darier's disease (Figure 4.18) and Hailey-Hailey disease. However the former is usu-ally associated with longitudinal erythronychia and subungual keratosis.
- Transverse leuconychia that may be monodactylous (single trauma, liquid nitrogen on the proximal nail fold or

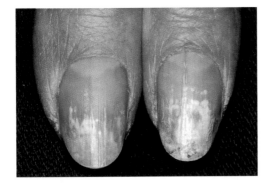

Figure 4.15

Nail varnish keratin granulations.

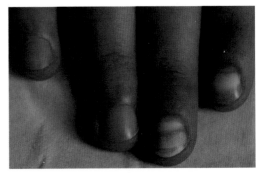

Figure 4.17

Congenital transverse leuconychia.

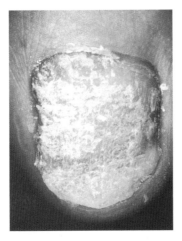

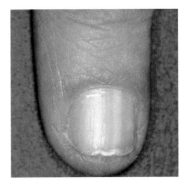

Figure 4.18

Darier's disease.

Figure 4.16

Psoriasis.

febrile infectious diseases and erythema multiforme), or polydactylous (excessive manicure); it may also be due to repeated microtrauma to untrimmed toenails (Figure 4.19).

- Psoriatic transverse leuconychia (Figure 4.20) is often accompanied by pitting of the nail and oil droplets.
- Neurological disorders such as sympathetic reflex dystrophy, C4 spinal cord injury, etc.

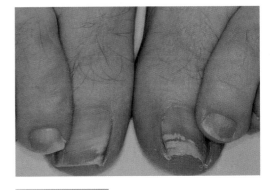

Figure 4.19

Mechanical transverse leuconychia.

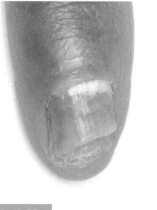

Figure 4.20

Transverse leuconychia due to psoriasis.

- Arsenic (Mees' bands), thallium and, much more often, drug reactions due to cytotoxic agents, where each session produces a polydactylous transverse line.
- Apparent leuconychia has to be differentiated from cirrhotic nail (where the whitening extends to 1–2 mm from the distal edge of the nail); the uraemic half-and-half nail (two segments separated transversally by a well-defined line); and Muehrcke's lines, mainly seen in hypoalbuminaemia (they run parallel to the lunula and are separated from one another and from the lunula by strikes of pink nail).
- Anaemia may produce pallor if the haemoglobin level falls sufficiently.

Proximal subungual onychomycosis with paronychia

This type of fungal infection can be mimicked by any factor that causes

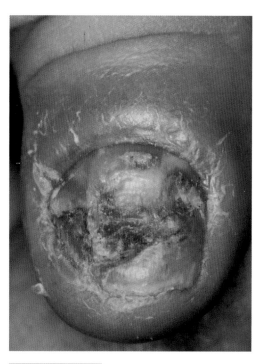

Figure 4.21

Parakeratosis pustulosa (Hjorth-Sabouraud disease).

paronychia with subsequent nail dystrophy (Figure 4.21, Table 4.2).

Fungal melanonychia (Figures 4.22–4.25, Table 4.3)

Haematoma, subungual tumours, foreign bodies, longitudinal melanonychia (Figure 4.26) and even malignant melanoma (Figure 4.27) should be ruled out. Dermoscopy examination of any blackish nail is the first step in reaching the proper diagnosis before excisional biopsy.[14]

TABLE 4.2	Main causes of chronic or subacute paronychia

Infective
- bacterial
  - staphylococci, streptococci
  - *Pseudomonas, Proteus mirabilis*
  - syphilis
- viral
  - herpes
  - warts (beneath the proximal nail fold)
- parasitic (tungiasis)

Dermatological
- contact dermatitis
- parakeratosis pustulosa (Figure 4.21)
- psoriasis, Reiter'syndrome
- ingrowing toenail
- pemphigus
- Darier's disease

Drugs
- antiretroviral drugs
- cytotoxic drugs
- retinoids

Microtrauma
- manicure

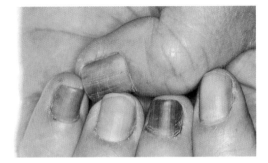

Figure 4.22

Fungal melanonychia due to *Candida guilliermondii.*

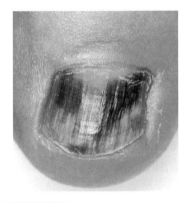

Figure 4.23

Fungal melanonychia due to *T. rubrum nigricans.*

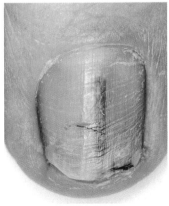

Figure 4.24

T. rubrum nigricans onychomycosis presenting as longitudinal melanonychia.

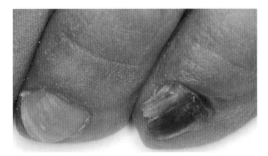

Figure 4.25

Frictional melanchonychia.

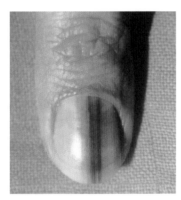

Figure 4.26

Acromelanoma.

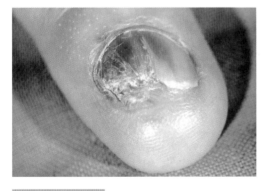

Figure 4.27

Malignant melanoma.

TABLE 4.3	Fungal causes of melanonychia (some of these fungi may be only possible causative organisms)

Acrothecium nigrum[4]
Aureobasidium pullulans
Alternaria grisea
Candida albicans
Candida humicola[5]
Candida tropicalis
Chaetomium globosum[6]
Chaetomium kunze
Chaetomium perpulchrum
Cladophialophora carrionii
Cladosporium sphaerospermum
Curvularia lunata
Fusarium oxysporum[7]
Hormodendrum elatum[6]
Phyllostictina sydowi
Pyrenochaeta unguis-hominis
Scopulariopsis brumptii[6]
Scytalidium dimidiatum (Natrassia mangifera, Hendersonula toruloidea)
T. mentagrophytes var. *mentagrophytes*[8]
Trichophyton rubrum[9–12]
Trichophyton soudanense
Wangiella dermatitidis[13]

References

1. Baran R, Dawber RPR, de Berker RPR, Haneke E, Tosti A. Diseases of the Nails and their Management, 3rd edn. Oxford, Blackwell Science, 2001

2. Zaias N. The Nail in Health and Disease, 2nd edn. Norwalk, CT, Lange & Appleton, 1990

3. Scher R. Nails, Therapy, Diagnosis, Surgery. Philadelphia, WB Saunders, 1990

4. Young WJ. Pigmented mycotic growth beneath the nail. Arch Dermatol 1934; 30:186

5. Velez A, Fernandez-Roldan JC. Melanonychia due to *Candida humicola*. Br J Dermatol 1996; 134:375–6

6. Tanuma H. Current topics in diagnosis and treatment of tinea unguium in Japan J Dermatol 1999; 26:87–90

7. Ritchie EB, Pinkerton ME. *Fusarium oxysporum* infection of the nail. Arch Dermatol 1959; 79:705

8. Soares Ribeiro LH, Maya TC, Piñero Macera J et al. Melanoniquia estriada: estudio de tres casos e analise comparativa da bibliografía pesquisada. Anal Bras Dermatol 1998; 73:341–4

9. Badillet G, Panagiotidou D, Sené S. Etude rétrospective des *Trichophyton rubrum* à pigment noir diffusible isolés à Paris de 1971 à 1980. Bull Soc Fr Mycol Med 1984; 13:117–20

10. Badillet G. Mélanonychies superficielles. Bull Soc Fr Mycol Med 1988; 17:335–40.

11. Higashi N. Melanonychia due to tinea unguium. Hifu 1990; 32:379–80

12. Perrin C, Baran R. Longitudinal melanonychia caused by *Trichophyton rubrum*. Histochemical and ultrastructural study of two cases. J Am Acad Dermatol 1994; 31:311–16

13. Matsumoto T, Matsudea T, Padhye AA et al. Fungal melanonychia: an ungual phaeohyphomycosis caused by *Wangiella dermatitidis*. Clin Exp Dermatol 1992; 17:83–6

14. Baran R, Dawber RPR, Haneke E, Tosti A, Bristow I. A Text Atlas of Nail Disorders. London, Taylor & Francis, 2003

Mycological examination

The clinical patterns seen in fungal nail disease only provide a clue to the type of infection. Although certain types of nail involvement are characteristic of certain species, usually the clinical appearance caused by one species of fungus is indistinguishable from that caused by another. Therefore, the diagnosis of onychomycosis always requires laboratory confirmation. Mycological diagnosis of onychomycosis is based on detection of fungal elements in KOH or tetraethyl ammonium hydroxide preparations of the nail samples, histopathology and identification of the responsible fungus by culture.[1-6] However, this may sometimes be difficult as fungi are not always isolated from nails due to their low number and viability. False negative mycological results are quite common, especially when samples are taken from a distal nail clipping. Negative mycology does not therefore completely rule out onychomycosis, since direct microscopy may be negative in up to 20% of cases and cultures may fail to isolate a fungus in up to 30% of cases. Recent treatment with topical antifungals may increase the risk of a false negative culture.

Therefore, when the clinical features strongly suggest onychomycosis, it is advisable to perform microscopic examination and culture more than once if initial investigations are negative. This is also recommended when the KOH preparation is positive and cultures are negative.

On the other hand, isolation of a fungus from a nail sample does not necessarily indicate onychomycosis. Saprophytic fungi will colonize the nail and may be cultured from nail samples. Therefore laboratory results should always be carefully evaluated and it is very important to correlate the clinical findings with the mycological findings. The clinician must always bear in mind that some fungi such as yeasts and most non-dermatophytic moulds are nail saprophytes rather than pathogens.

A correct diagnosis of onychomycosis depends on several factors including accuracy of specimen collection, expertise of the laboratory staff and skill in the evaluation of the laboratory results. The application of molecular mycological diagnostic techniques is at an early stage and it is not possible to evaluate this approach at present.

A glossary of terms is shown in Table 5.1.

TABLE 5.1	Glossary of terms

Conidia: asexual spores
Dematiaceous: brown-black pigmented fungus
Dermatophytes: filamentous fungi specialized in the digestion of keratin
Floccose: fluffy, cottony
Hyphae: branching filaments formed by a chain of cells
Mycelium: mass of hyphae
Moulds: filamentous fungi
Phialide: a conidiogenous cell that produces a succession of blastic conidia without increasing in length
Spores: reproductive cells
Yeasts: unicellular budding fungi

How and where to collect the samples properly

Correct collection of the specimen is essential in order to avoid false negative results as well as to eliminate contaminants (Figure 5.1). The site of specimen sampling depends on the clinical type of onychomycosis. It is always important to collect as much material as possible, as the nail may contain only a few fungal elements. Separate samples should be obtained from fingernails and toenails. Since toenail onychomycosis is frequently associated with tinea pedis, it is best to collect samples for mycology not only from the nails, but also from the soles. The same rule applies for the palms of patients with fingernail onychomycosis.

Distal subungual onychomycosis

Samples should be obtained from the nail bed and ventral nail plate. It is very important to try to collect material from the most proximal portion of the affected nail bed. This is the area most likely to contain viable fungi. The affected nail bed is exposed by removing the overlying onycholytic nail plate with a nail clipper; then appropriate material is taken by scraping the hyperkeratotic nail bed with a solid or disposable scalpel or a curette (Figure 5.2).

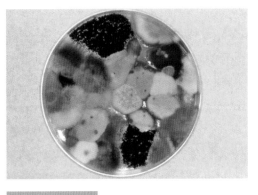

Figure 5.1

Growth of contaminants from a distal nail clipping.

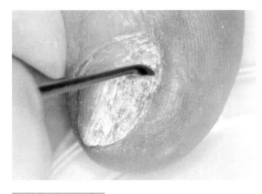

Figure 5.2

Collection of specimens from a nail affected by distal subungual onychomycosis. Subungual scales are obtained with a curette after removal of the onycholytic nail plate.

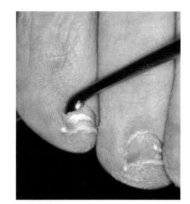

Figure 5.3

Collection of specimens from a nail affected by white superficial onychomycosis. The leuconychial area is directly scraped with a curette.

It is advisable, where possible, not to include the distal nail plate in the sample, since it frequently contains contaminants that may obscure the growth of pathogenic fungi.

White superficial onychomycosis/black superficial onychomycosis

Samples should be obtained from the friable areas of leuconychia (or melanonychia) of the superficial nail plate. Shallow shaving with a disposable scalpel or gentle scraping of the dorsum of the nail with a curette will provide specimens for microscopy and culture (Figure 5.3).

Proximal subungual onychomycosis

Samples should be obtained from the intermediate nail plate The affected nail plate is exposed by perforating the proximal nail with a disposable punch or an electric drill (Figure 5.4). The latter procedure offers the advantage of avoiding the necessity for anaesthesia and the risk of bleeding. Scales are then obtained by scraping the exposed nail plate with a disposable scalpel.

Chronic paronychia

Samples can be taken from beneath the proximal nail fold by passing a disposable loop under the affected area of the fold, but the presence of *Candida* alone should not be interpreted as an indication that it is the only factor involved in causing the disease.

Endonyx onychomycosis

Viable fungi are present throughout the whole thickness of the nail plate. Nail clippings can therefore be used for mycology.

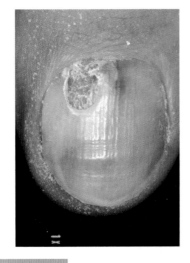

Figure 5.4

Collection of specimens in a case of proximal subungual onychomycosis. Scales are collected from the intermediate nail after perforation of the nail plate with a disposable punch.

Microscopic examination

After collection, specimens are placed in a Petri dish or in a dark envelope or mailing pack and sent to the laboratory. Immediate examination is not mandatory since fungi remain viable in nail specimens for several months.

Before examination, the nail material is divided into small fragments; half of the sample is usually used for direct microscopy and the other half for culture. Thick materials need to be pulverized; this can be achieved by crushing the nail specimens with a hammer or using a nail micronizer.

The nail material is placed on a glass slide with a drop of 20–30% KOH. After apply-

ing a coverslip, gently heating the slide in a Bunsen flame accelerates clearing of the keratin and allows visualization of the fungal elements. The coverslip is then gently pushed down with a pencil to flatten the scales. Screening should be carried out as soon as possible to avoid deterioration of the specimen.

Using 20% KOH in a vehicle of 60% water and 40% DMSO provides a more rapid method of diagnosis of mycosis without heating, and the specimens last longer for re-examination.

Identification of fungi may be facilitated by adding a drop of chlorazol black E (Sigma), a counter-stain specific for chitin, to the KOH preparation. Only the fungal elements develop a greenish-blue colour and chlorazol black E may help to differentiate these from artifacts. Alternatively the hyphae can be stained with a fluorochrome (calcofluor white) but this requires a fluorescence microscope. It is, however, a very accurate method of screening nails.

The microscope is set with the condenser in a low position and the diaphragm is shut down so as to produce a dark background that contrasts with the light-refracting hyphae. The slide is first screened at low power (10× objective). Details can be discerned using the 40× objective. Fungal hyphae appear as elongated branching, septate, light-refracting structures that pass across the horny cells (Figure 5.5). It is impossible to differentiate non-viable from viable fungi.

Fungal elements should be differentiated from artifacts including lipid vesicles, air bubbles, textile fibres and mosaic fun-

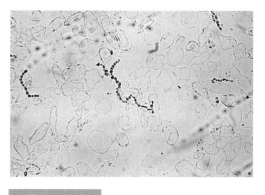

Figure 5.5

Potassium hydroxide (KOH) preparation of a nail sample showing refractial branching hyphae.

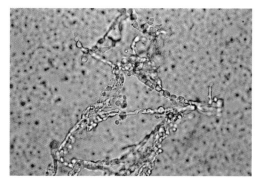

Figure 5.6

KOH preparation of a *Scopulariopsis brevicaulis* nail infection. Elongated branching hyphae together with lemon-shaped conidia characteristic of this fungus are shown.

gus. The latter is a common artefact caused by lipid deposition at the periphery of the host cells.

Microscopic examination can differentiate yeast cells from dermatophyte hyphae and other moulds, but species identification cannot be made from wet mounts. However, *Scopulariopsis brevicaulis* may be identified when thick-walled, pigmented lemon-shaped spores are seen (Figure 5.6), and *Scytalidium dimidiatum* and *S. hyalinum* can be suspected by their narrow tortuous hyphae.

Since different causative organisms may require different therapies, reliable identification of the causal agent is important and this can only be made by culture.

Culture

Half of the specimen should be set up for culture even when microscopic examination is negative.

In order to grow both dermatophytes and non-dermatophytes it is always important to inoculate the material into two different media :

1. Sabouraud glucose-agar with 0.05% chloramphenicol that permits the growth of dermatophytes, non-dermatophytes and yeasts.
2. Sabouraud glucose-agar with 0.05% chloramphenicol and 0.4% cyclo-heximide (Actidione®), which allows the growth of dermatophytes, but inhibits the growth of yeasts and most non-dermatophytic moulds.

Inoculation is carried out using a sterile needle and 10–20 pieces of specimen are gently pushed into each medium. Cultures are incubated at 24–28°C. Non-dermatophytic moulds grow faster than dermatophytes and produce well-formed colonies within 1 week. Colonies of most dermatophytes are usually completely differentiated in 2 weeks. A negative result is the absence of growth after 3–6 weeks. All plates should be kept for a minimum of 2 weeks in case mould or yeast growth obscures that of a dermatophyte.

Identification of the fungus is based on growth rate and the macroscopic and microscopic appearance of the colony. For this purpose, a small portion of the colony is selected by pressing a strip of sellotape onto the surface of the culture. The tape is then placed on a slide and stained with lactophenol cotton blue. Alternatively, pieces of colony can be teased out with a sterile needle.

Media containing a phenol red pH indicator that changes from yellow to red in the presence of dermatophytes are also available on the market (DTM) (Figure 5.7). These media contain antibiotics and cycloheximide to inhibit contaminant bacteria and fungi. However, some contaminants can still grow in the

medium and produce a red discoloration that can be erroneously interpreted as a sign of dermatophyte growth. Although routine use of these media is not recommended, they can be helpful when laboratory facilities are not available.

Table 5.2 shows the main organisms that cause onychomycosis.

Dermatophytes

T. rubrum – Within 2 weeks *T. rubrum* forms dome-shaped floccose white colonies with a well defined dark red-brown to yellow reverse (Figures 5.8 and 5.9).

Lactophenol cotton blue mounts of the colonies show sparse club-shaped microconidia along the sides of the hyphae.

T. mentagrophytes var. *interdigitale* – Within 2 weeks *T. interdigitale* forms powdery white colonies with a cream centre and a pale to dark-brown reverse (Figure 5.10).

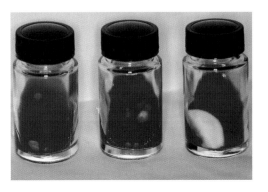

Figure 5.7

Proof of growth of dermatophytes (DTM). In case of growth the medium changes its colour to red.

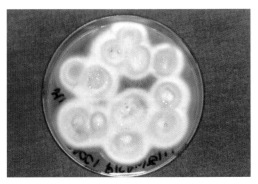

Figure 5.8

Trichophyton rubrum. Macroscopic appearance of the colony.

TABLE 5.2	Causes of onychomycosis	
COMMON		**UNCOMMON**
	Dermatophytes	
T. rubrum		*Epidermophyton floccosum*
T. mentagrophytes var. *interdigitale*		*T. soudanense*
		T. violaceum
		T. mentagrophytes var. *mentagrophytes*
		M. canis
		T. tonsurans
		T. erinacei
		T. equinum
		M. gypseum
	Moulds	
Scopulariopsis brevicaulis		*Acremonium* spp.
Fusarium spp.		*Aspergillus* spp.
		Scytalidium spp.
		Onychocola canadensis
		Chaetomium globosum
		Paecilomyces spp.
	Yeasts	
		Candida albicans
		Candida parapsilosis

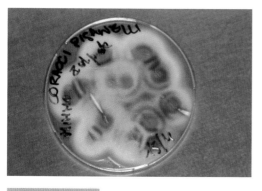

Figure 5.9

The reverse appearance of Figure 5.8 2 weeks after inoculation.

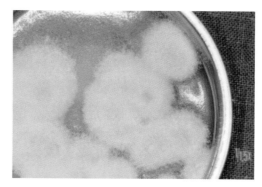

Figure 5.10

Trichophyton interdigitale. Macroscopic appearance of the colony 2 weeks after inoculation.

Lactophenol cotton blue mounts of the colonies reveal abundant microconidia along the sides and at the ends of branched hyphae (Figure 5.11). Characteristic spiral hyphae may be present.

Non-dermatophyte moulds

Non-dermatophyte moulds are widespread in the environment as soil and plant saprophytes, and can frequently be found in the nails as contaminants. Isolating a non-dermatophyte mould from nail material does not necessarily have any pathological significance and the results of cultures should always be correlated with the nail signs. In particular, non-dermatophyte moulds are commonly isolated from toenails affected by traumatic onycholysis, onychogryphosis and pachyonychia, where they are present as saprophytes.

Laboratory diagnosis of non-dermatophyte mould onychomycosis requires the following criteria:[7]

- presence of hyphae in the KOH preparation; sometimes these are irregular in shape or are pigmented.
- growth of the fungus in at least five inocula on the same plate.
- isolation of the same mould from three consecutive nail samples.

Scopulariopsis brevicaulis – *Scopulariopsis brevicaulis* grows in media both with and without cycloheximide. Within 1 week it forms brown colonies with powdery surfaces and pale brown reverse (Figure 5.12).

Lactophenol cotton blue mounts of the colonies reveal numerous branched conidiophores with chains of lemon-shaped conidia.

Fusarium **spp.** Growth of *Fusarium* spp. requires cycloheximide-free medium.

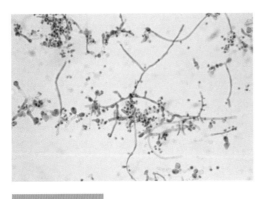

Figure 5.11

Lactophenol cotton blue mount of a colony of *Trichophyton interdigitale*. Abundant round mitoconidia along the sides and the ends of branched hyphae are shown.

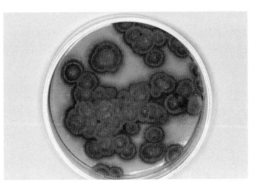

Figure 5.12

Scopulariopsis brevicaulis. Macroscopic appearance of the colony 2 weeks after inoculation.

Within a week *Fusarium* spp. produce flat colonies which are pale pink or brownish in colour (Figure 5.13).

Culture mounts in lactophenol cotton blue show numerous sickle-shaped macroconidia and elliptical and oval microconidia. These arise from short phialidic cells in colonies of *Fusarium oxysporum*, or long phialidic cells in colonies of *Fusarium solani*.

***Aspergillus* spp.** – Growth of *Aspergillus* spp. requires cycloheximide-free medium. The macroscopic appearance of the colonies varies among the different species.

Lactophenol cotton blue mounts of the colonies are diagnostic due to the typical vesiculate heads and conidial chains.

***Acremonium* spp.** – *Acremonium* spp. grow in media both with and without cycloheximide. In cycloheximide-free medium *Acremonium* forms white-pink velvety colonies within 1 week.

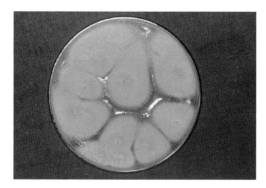

Fusarium solani. Macroscopic appearance of the colony 1 week after inoculation.

Lactophenol cotton blue mounts of the colonies reveal elliptical conidia grouped at the tips of long phialides. They can be confused with *Fusarium* spp.

***Scytalidium* spp.** – In cycloheximide-free medium, *Scytalidum* spp. produce fast-growing colonies with an abundant aerial mycelium that, in some cultures, fills a Petri dish within a few days. Others are slower. Colonies of *Scytalidium dimidiatum* are initially white and become black or dark brown in a few days, while colonies of *Scytalidium hyalinum* remain white or creamy in colour.

Lactophenol cotton blue mounts of the colonies reveal the chains of arthro-spores, which are brown-walled in the colonies of *Scytalidium dimidiatum*.

Histopathological examination

Virchow (1855) was the first to give a detailed histopathological description of dermatophyte-infected nails.[8] Particular histopathological patterns of infection were described later, mostly on avulsed nails,[9–20] rarely on nail biopsies.[21–26] Until very recently virtually all mycologists and many dermatologists claimed that direct microscopy using KOH-cleared specimens and mycological cultures are the gold standard of diagnostic measures for skin and nail mycoses. Histological methods were only used by few researchers who had great difficulties in defending histopathology as a supplementary diagnostic method and valuable research tool. Now histopathology is on the way to being accepted as an important diagnostic aid.[27–38] It has its undoubted advantages and has repeatedly been reported to be clearly superior to the routine mycological diagnostic procedures in terms of sensitivity and in part also specificity.[24,29,30] The results of histopathological examinations are obtained much faster than culture – usually 1–3 days versus 3 or more weeks.[24,26] Histopathology is much more often positive than cultures.[15,24,26,30,35] In a series of 400 consecutive patients with onychomycosis-suggestive nail changes, fungi were found twice as often histologically as compared with culture.[30] The method also shows whether there are hyphae and/or spores, whether the fungal organisms grow as invasive filamentous pathogens in the nail plate and/or in the subungual hyperkeratosis, how the nail is damaged by the pathogenic fungi, and whether there are pits and abundant parakeratosis in addition to intracorneal polymorphonuclear leukocytes suggesting psoriasis.[24,26,39]

Histopathology of nail clippings

Histopathology of clipped nail specimens from onychomycoses has gained increased acceptance in the last 10–15 years.[26–38] The nail plate material should preferably contain as much subungual debris as possible. In more than 90% of cases, PAS staining is sufficient for the diagnosis – confirmation or exclusion of onychomycosis. Enrichment of the specimen using KOH-treated nail clippings stained with PAS (the KONCPA technique) may further enhance the sensitivity of histopathology,[40] although this could not be confirmed in another study comparing conventional PAS staining with KONCPA, fluorescent whitening agents and KONCFLU (KOH-treated nail

clippings treated with fluorescent whitening agents).[41] Additional stains like Grocott's and Gridley's may be used; however, they very rarely give a positive result when PAS was negative. In addition, they use the same chemical residues to stain fungal elements as PAS and thus do not really increase the accuracy of differential diagnosis against PAS-positive non-fungal structures.[24,26,42] Blancophores (fluorescent whitening agents) are even more specific. This fluorescent dye specifically stains fungal cell walls because of their chitin content; chitin is a typical constituent of fungal cell walls and does not exist in vertebrates. Therefore, in contrast to PAS and Grocott, blancophore does not stain serum remnants, which may be compressed between keratinocytes and onychocytes and may look very much like fungal filaments in PAS-stained sections, and neither PAS- nor Grocott-positive neutrophil leukocytes are stained. However, textile fibres stain very intensely but stand out because of their extremely bright fluorescence.[42]

Nail plate should be processed for histopathology without prior formalin fixation; where there is abundant subungual debris, short formalin fixation is recommended because this material is not dry like the nail plate and often contains saprophytic bacteria that are able to live on and degrade keratin. However, the keratin material may be immersed in 10% urea solution overnight to make it softer and easier to section. Another possibility is to fix it in 3% phenol to soften the nail keratin. The clippings are embedded in paraffin or paraplast, cut into 4–6 μ sections and stained with haematoxylin and eosin (H&E) as well as with PAS. Sectioning of nail specimens, mounting of the sections without folding, and staining without floating off the sections requires a lot of experience on the part of the technicians.[24,26,42]

Nail plate material can be obtained by clipping as much of the distal nail plate as possible, the clipping preferably reaching to the border between the fungal infection and the healthy nail. Often there is a thick infected toenail plate that, after removal, reveals considerable keratotic debris on the nail bed. This should also be taken for the histopathological examination. Clippings are useful in cases of distal–lateral subungual onychomycosis and for the so-called yellow streak (yellow spike) or dermatophytoma. Different nail clippers, an English nail splitter, sturdy straight scissors or special toenail scissors with a long handle and very short cutting edges may be used. For superficial white onychomycosis, a layer of the dorsal surface of the nail plate may be cut tangentially from the nail using a #23 or #15 scalpel. Proximal white subungual onychomycosis very often demonstrates proximal onycholysis, thus allowing a punch biopsy to be taken from the nail plate without prior anaesthesia. The nail is softened with a 10-minute warm finger or foot bath and a disposable 4-mm punch is used to cut out a disc of nail plate. Immediately prior to reaching the nail bed with the sharp punch the patient will feel the sharp instrument and say when to stop. The little disc of nail may be cut into two halves, one for histopathology, the other for mycological culture.[42] In cases of suspected endonyx onychomycosis, as much of the nail plate is clipped as is possible

without hurting the patient too much. In total dystrophic onychomycosis, it is usually easy to cut away large chunks of the infected nail material.

Histopathology of nail plate specimens varies according to the clinical type of onychomycosis, the severity of the nail changes and the abundance of fungi in and under the nail. As is known from mycological cultures, subungual keratinous debris commonly contains more fungal elements than the plate itself (Figure 5.14). In the nail, fungal hyphae are usually found in the under-surface of the nail plate. Fine filaments are arranged in a longitudinal direction, often remarkably parallel, which is a sign of a hitherto undisturbed nail growth. Depending on the severity, they may be seen as slender, septate hyphae in a compact nail plate or as thick, septate elements showing shorter and longer intersections as well as relatively large round spores. The latter are seen to have a basophilic content in H&E stains and are probably dermatophyte arthrospores (Figure 5.15). Subungual keratinous material may be adherent to the nail plate and contain very large amounts of short thick hyphae and spores. They may invade the nail plate causing splits as well as vertical and branching defects in the deep nail plate layers. Quite often, the thick subungual hyperkeratosis appears papillomatous and contains large globules of dried serum (Figure 5.14) as well as intracorneal neutrophils morphologically indistinguishable from Munro's microabscesses; however, there is usually much less parakeratosis in onychomycosis than in ungual psoriasis. Fungal filaments are also seen in close

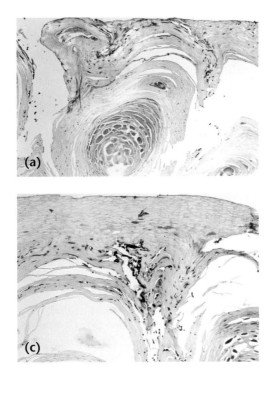

(a)

(c)

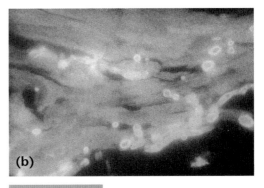

(b)

Figure 5.14

(a) Undersurface of nail plate and subungual hyperkeratosis containing abundant slender hyphae of *Trichophyton rubrum* as well as PAS positive serum inclusions. Half polarized light, PAS, magnification ×100. (b) Undersurface of nail plate containing fungal filaments and spores. Blancophore fluorochrome magnification ×250. (c) Distal subungual onychomycosis with masses of hyphae in the deep nail plate layer and arthrospores in a nail split. PAS, magnification ×100.

vicinity to serum inclusions, although dermatophytes are presumed not to grow in the presence of serum (Figure 5.14a). Subungual debris clinically appearing as relatively soft material often contains huge numbers of large, thick-walled, polyhedral spores between horny cells; however, they may germinate and form short thick filaments penetrating the nail plate (Figure 5.15). They may be non-dermatophyte moulds, but histopathology cannot confirm this with absolute certainty because dermatophytes may also form large arthrospores sometimes with outgrowth of short thick-walled hyphae.[24,26,42] The clinical phenomenon of a yellow longitudinal stripe, which is often seen in dermatophytic toenail infections, shows abundant large spores and short filaments compressed in a tube-like space formed by the overlying nail plate and subungual keratin. Because of the huge masses of compressed fungal elements the term 'dermatophytoma' was coined.[43] Even by light microscopy, the extremely thick walls of the fungal elements can be

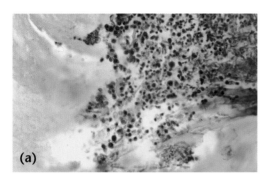

(a)

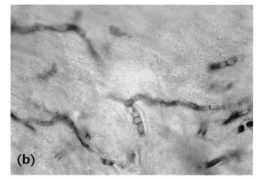

(b)

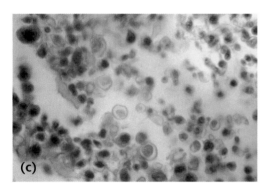

(c)

Figure 5.15

Huge masses of spores and a few short hyphae are seen in deep nail plate layers. (a) Undersurface of nail plate with fungi and serum globules. PAS, magnification ×250. (b) Branched septate hyphae are seen in nail plate above the spores. PAS, magnfication ×400. (c) Large spores are situated in nail plate defect. PAS, magnification ×400.

discerned. However, *Scopulariopsis brevicaulis*, particularly in the great toenail of elderly women, also forms large fungal masses in the line of the nail bed ridges that proceed proximally, eventually merge and give rise to a typical yellow to yellowish-brown streak.[9,17,44] *Scopulariopsis brevicaulis* can often be identified by its lemon-shaped polygonal shape. Chromomycoses seen in tropical regions may be diagnosed with H&E stains as large round to oval brown spores in the keratin of the nail bed. Cultural identification is advisable.

In superficial onychomycosis, either chains of regularly sized small spores can be seen in splits of the nail plate surface (Figure 5.16a) or short hyphae and spores have invaded the surface layers (Figure 5.16b). No inflammatory cells are seen (Figure 5.16). Non-dermatophyte mould infections can cause the clinical aspect of superficial white onychomycosis but invade the nail plate deeper,[38,45] but this is also seen in *Trichophyton rubrum* nail infections of AIDS patients.[45]

Punched segments of nail plate from proximal white subungual onychomycosis usually show a compact nail plate without inflammatory cells. Different layers of the entire thickness of the plate are invaded by large amounts of fungal filaments that are arranged longitudinally and in a parallel manner. Almost total nail plate invasion was also seen in a case of *Candida albicans* proximal onychomycosis in a newborn (unpublished observation).

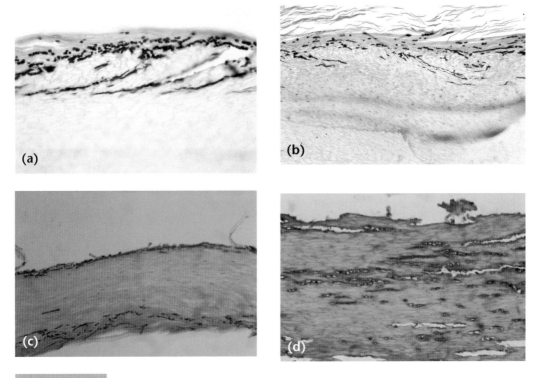

(a) (b) (c) (d)

Superficial white onychomycosis. (a) Chains of regular small spores of *Trichophyton mentagrophytes* in SWO. Nail biopsy, PAS, magnification ×250. (b) Short fungal hyphae and spores in SWO of an AIDs patient. PAS, magnification ×100. (c) Superficial and ventral fungal invasion: bipolar type. PAS, magnification ×100. (d) 'Deep' superficial onychomycosis with massive fungal invasion of the nail plate, PAS, magnification ×250.

In total dystrophic onychomycosis, only small nail plate fragments are left or large masses of irregular hyperkeratoses overlie the nail field. Nail plate remnants with keratotic debris show variable amounts of fungal elements that are haphazardly arranged, in contrast to distal and proximal subungual onychomycosis with their parallel arrangement of fungal hyphae. In addition to yeast cells, filamentous fungal elements may some-times be seen. There are also inflammatory cells and serum inclusions.[42]

Histopathology of nail biopsies

Nail biopsies are not commonly required to make the diagnosis of distal subungual onychomycosis, but they are powerful tools for research and may be the only means of differentiating onychomycosis from nail psoriasis, lichen planus, alopecia areata, nail eczema, and other inflammatory nail disorders.[39] A ring-block anaesthesia at the base of the digit or a transthecal anaesthesia for a long finger are recommended. If there is a large area of onycholysis and/or a considerable amount of subungual debris, perioperative antibiotic prophylaxis may be wise. A surgical scrub is recommended on the evening and the morning prior to nail biopsy and thorough repeated disinfection is necessary immediately before, during and after the procedure. It is worth noting that in this case no material for cultures can be taken from the biopsied nail organ because the disinfective agent will prevent growth of the microorganisms. Usually, a lateral longitudinal nail biopsy is taken yielding a 2-mm wide block of tissue containing the entire length of the nail plate with overlying proximal nail fold, underlying matrix and nail bed as well as hyponychium and adjacent skin of the tip of the digit. Care has to be taken not to shear the nail plate off its underlying structures in order to allow the correct anatomical relationships to be visualized. The tissue is fixed in 5% formalin or 3% phenol[46] and processed as usual. Before cutting sections the block is oriented and a drop of 20–40% KOH solution is laid on its surface to soften the nail plate component of the tissue specimen; this is done to avoid accidental shearing of the hard nail plate from the ungual soft tissues during sectioning.

The histopathology of biopsies of the nail apparatus including the proximal nail fold, matrix, nail bed and hyponychium confirms the findings described above from nail clippings, but also gives information about the involvement of the ungual soft tissues that are responsible for nail formation and growth, attachment to the nail bed and the nail's appearance.

Longitudinal biopsies from cases of distal subungual onychomycosis show essentially the same type of alterations in the nail plate and adherent keratosis as seen in nail clippings. The nail bed develops subungual hyperkeratosis that initially covers the distal portion of the nail bed but progresses proximally toward the matrix with time. It contains abundant hyphae, quite frequently large amounts of serum inclusions and often also pycnotic neutrophils and a few lymphocytes. The neutrophils may form typical intracorneal spongiform abscesses which, however, are usually situated within predominantly orthokeratotic hyperkeratoses. The more severe the onychomycosis the more proximally these changes will have advanced. The nail plate itself is only invaded in its lower layers. The fungi are seen to lie in a longitudinal parallel arrangement. The nail bed epithelium often exhibits considerable spongiosis with lymphocytic exocytosis and only few intermingled neutrophils. There may be a dense mononuclear inflammatory infiltrate in the upper dermis with some accentuation perivascularly. When distal subungual onychomycosis secondarily progresses to total dystrophic onychomycosis, nail bed and matrix alterations become more pronounced. The epithelium may become papillomatous, heavily oedematous and infiltrated with neutrophils and/or lymphocytes. Pseudobullous subepithelial oedema may develop. The distal nail plate breaks away but the proximal third under the proximal nail fold usually remains more or less intact.[24]

Superficial white onychomycosis shows the same picture in nail biopsies as in clippings or shave biopsies. There is no inflammatory infiltrate in the nail bed beneath the fungal invasion and the nail bed and matrix remain normal[24] (Figure 5.3).

Endonyx onychomycosis has been observed due to *T. soudanense* or *T. violaceum* infection. Large amounts of hyphae are seen in the nail plate virtually without involvement of the nail bed. Inflammatory changes are practically absent, although there may be a slight nail bed hyperkeratosis (Figure 5.17).[25,32,47]

Proximal (white) subungual onychomycosis shows some fungal filaments in the stratum corneum of the under-surface of the proximal nail fold. From here, fungi may also invade the nail plate surface

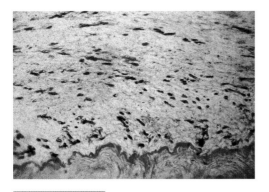

Figure 5.17

Endonyx onychomycosis. PAS, magnification ×250.

(Figure 5.18) which may give rise to the picture of superficial white onychomycosis growing out from under the nail fold[24] (Figure 5.16a). This has recently been confirmed by a histopathological study.[37] There is only a sparse inflammatory reaction to the fungal infection of the eponychium. The pathogens slowly progress toward the proximal end of the matrix. When the latter is reached the relatively fast-growing matrix cells differentiating into onychocytes will incorporate the fungi and transport them distally and away from the matrix epithelium while the nail plate grows out. Part of the fungus further progresses along the matrix–nail plate junction in a distal direction toward the nail bed. All along the matrix, fungal elements are continuously included into the growing nail plate and thus transported away from the matrix until the nail bed is reached. This is the reason for the minimal inflammatory response to the infection in the matrix area over a long period of time. It also explains why in this particular form of nail infection, fungi may be found in all layers of the nail plate. Only late in the course of proximal subungual onychomycosis will the matrix respond with inflammatory changes similar to those described for the nail bed; then the nail plate will no longer be formed in a regular way and total dystrophic onychomycosis will soon develop. When the fungi arrive at the nail bed they induce a reaction similar to that seen in distal subungual onychomycosis with nail bed hyperkeratosis and inflammation.[24] A case of proximal subungual onychomycosis due to *Candida albicans* was described in a boy with recurrent chronic mucocutaneous candidosis.[48]

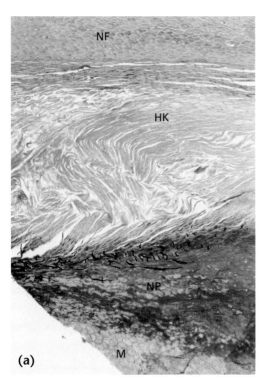

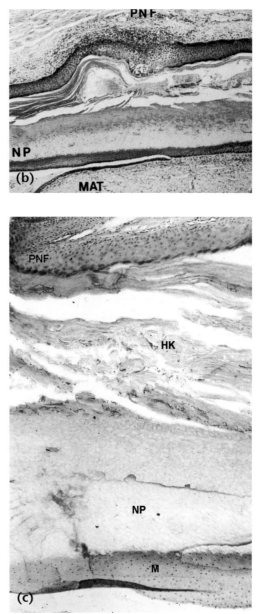

Figure 5.18

Proximal subungual onychomycosis. (a) Marked hyperkeratosis (HK) of the ventral surface of the proximal nail fold (NF) and fungal filaments in the nail plate (NP). M, matrix. Nail biopsy. Grocott, magnification ×100. (b) Fungal invasion of the hyperkeratosis of PNF undersurface (eponychium), dense lymphocytic infiltrate, focal spongiosis and exocytosis. (Image courtesy of N. Zaias, USA.) (c) Loose hyperkeratosis between the stratum corneum of the proximal nail fold's undersurface and the nail plate with fungal hyphae. Nail biopsy. PAS, magnfication ×100.

Total dystrophic onychomycosis, particularly in chronic mucocutaneous candidosis, shows a complete loss of an orderly nail structure. The proximal nail has receded to form a short rim of tissue (Figure 5.19a, b). Matrix and nail bed are papillomatous and hyperkeratotic with alternating hypergranulosis. Fungal filaments and spores irregularly penetrate the hyperkeratoses (Figure 5.19c, d). Electron microscopy shows candida spores and germ tubes. The matrix and nail bed epithelia respond with marked keratohyalin granule production and composite keratohyalin granules are abundant.[49] Exocytosis of lymphocytes is evident, with many of them exhibiting convoluted nuclei.[24,49]

Nail destruction by fungi

Histopathological examination of nail material also allows the study of the degree of nail dystrophy due to fungal invasion. A few spores scattered in splits of subungual keratin are probably just commensals. Large amounts of fungal organisms, whether filaments or spores, have to be considered pathogens. Commonly, spores and short thick hyphae are seen to lie in spaces of nail or subungual keratin. They often penetrate into the nail from beneath. The nail keratin next to the holes formed by the fungi often stains more eosinophilic, indicating chemical digestion. Very large amounts of fungi penetrating the entire thickness of the nail plate also reduce the mechanical resistance of the plate (Figure 5.15). Alkiewicz[9] described the transverse net which is a system of air-filled channels due to dermatophytes. A similar system of channels produced by dermatophyte digestion of nail keratin, but which is more confined to the matrix region, was described later.[50] *In vitro* investigations using electron microscopy have shown that invading dermatophyte and mould hyphae are both intra- and extra-cellular.[51]

Identification of fungi

Histopathology can distinguish between contaminants and pathogens, however, it cannot determine fungal species. Long slender hyphae are usually dermatophytes, but *Scytalidium dimidiatum* and *S. hyalinum* are similar. Short, branched, thick filaments are probably non-dermatophyte moulds. Dermatophytes can form huge amounts of thick-walled arthrospores also resembling non-dermatophyte moulds.[24,42] *Scopulariopsis brevicaulis* usually forms large polygonal spores.[52] *Candida albicans* may be identified by yeasts that form germ tubes, however, it may be difficult to differentiate true hyphae from pseudohyphae by light microscopy.[49]

Immunohistochemistry using polyclonal antibodies against pathogenetically relevant fungi, as well as flow cytometry, have been used to identify the pathogens of onychomycosis.[53] However, it has to be stressed that up to now, only mycological cultures are able to reliably identify the fungal pathogen.

In situ hybridization has not yet been successful in determining the fungal pathogens involved in onychomycosis because of lack of specific and sensitive primers.

PCR was initially disappointing, with not enough sensitive primers being

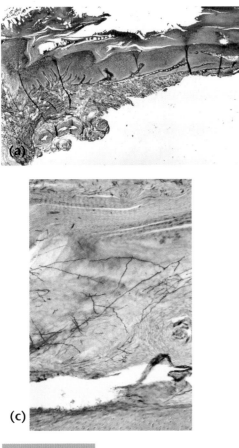

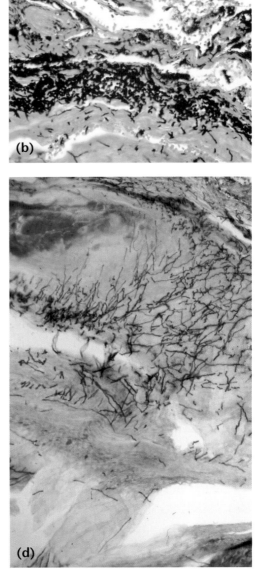

Figure 5.19

Total dystrophic onychomycosis.
(a) Primary total dystrophic onychomycosis in chronic mucocutaneous candidosis. Nail biopsy Grocott, magnification ×2.5.
(b) Primary total dystrophic onychomycosis in chronic mucocutaneous candidosis. Nail biopsy Grocott, magnification ×250.
(c) Total dystrophic onychomycosis secondary to distal subungual dermatophyte infection. PAS, magnification ×100. (d) Total dystrophic onychomycosis secondary to distal subungual onychomycosis. Haphazard arrangement of fungal filaments. PAS, magnification ×250.

available, but now has limited use in laboratory diagnosis.[54–58] However, although it is more sensitive and specific than culture it has the same disadvantage: it cannot distinguish between a pathogen and a contaminant, although this may one day be possible with *in situ* PCR-RT and PCR techniques.[59]

References

1. Midgley G, Moore MK, Cook JC et al. Mycology of nail disorders. J Am Acad Dermatol 1994; 31:568–74

2. Elewski BE. Clinical pearl: diagnosis of onychomycosis. J Am Acad Dermatol 1995; 32:500–1

3. Clayton Y, Midgley G. Medical Mycology. London, Gower Medical Publishing, 1985

4. Evans EGV, Richardson MD. Medical Mycology: A Medical Approach. Oxford, IRL Press, 1989

5. Campbell CK, Johnson EM, Philpot CM, Warnock DW. Identification of Pathogenic Fungi. London, Public Health Laboratory Service, 1996

6. Lasagni A. Atlante di Micologia. Milano, UTET Periodici Scientifici, 1996

7. English MP. Nails and fungi. Br J Dermatol 1976; 94:697–701

8. Virchow R. Zur normalen und pathologischen Anatomie der Nägel, insbesondere über hornige Entartung und Pilzbildung an den Nägeln. Verhandlungen der Würzburger medicinisch physicalischen Gesellschaft, 1855

9. Alkiewicz J. Transverse net in the diagnosis of onychomycosis. Arch Dermatol 1948; 58:385–9

10. Sagher F. Histologic examinations of fungous infections of the nails. J Invest Dermatol 1948; 11:337–57

11. Stühmer A. Subunguale Epidermophytie, Trichophytie und Favus. Eine bisher nicht bekannte Form von Nagelmykosen. Arch Dermatol Syph 1952; 193:527–36

12. Grimmer H. Histopathologie der Onychomyckose und ihre Bedeutung für die Griseofulvintherapie. Z Haut GeschlKr 1960; 28:365–8

13. Götz H. Pilzkrankheiten der Haut durch Dermatophyten. In Jadassohns Handbuch der Haut und Geschlechtskrankheiten, Ergänzungswerk vol IV/3. Heidelberg, Springer, 1960:350–1

14. Sowinski W. Trichophytic entrance sites into the nail in man. In Drouhet E, ed. CR Comm Ve Congr Int Mycol Hum Anim, Institut Pasteur, Paris, 1971

15. Bojanovsky A. Zur Bewertung des histologischen Nachweises von Onychomykosen. Castellania 1975; 3:169–71

16. Hauck H. Histologische Untersuchungen bei Nagelmykosen. 12th Scient Meet German Soc Mycol, Baden/Vienna, 1975, Book of Abstracts p. 7

17. Alkiewicz J, Pfister H. Atlas der Nagelkrankheiten. Pathohistologie, Klinik und Differentialdiagnose. New York, FK Schattauer, 1976

18. Achten G, Wanet-Rouard J. Onychomycoses in the laboratory. Mykosen 1978; Suppl 1:125–7

19. Scher RK, Ackerman AB. Subtle clues to diagnosis from biopsies of nails. Histologic differential diagnosis of onychomycosis and psoriasis of the nail unit from cornified cells of the nail bed alone. Am J Dermatopathol 1980; 2:255–6

20. Ho Ping Kong B, Kapica L, Lee R. Keratin invasion by *Hendersonula toruloidea*. A tropical pathogenic fungus resistant to therapy. Int J Dermatol 1984; 23:65–6

21. Zaias N. Onychomycosis. Arch Dermatol 1972; 105:263–74

22. Scher RK, Ackerman AB. Subtle clues to diagnosis from biopsies of nails. The value of nail biopsy for demonstrating fungi not demonstrable by microbiologic techniques. Am J Dermatopathol 1980; 2:55–7

23. Male O. Clinical significance of nail diseases. Nidaros Dermatol Soc, Trondheim, Norway, 1983

24. Haneke E. Nail biopsies in onychomycosis. Mykosen 1985; 28:473

25. Tosti A, Baran R, Piraccini MD, Fanti PA. "Endonyx" onychomycosis: a new modality

of nail invasion by dermatophytes. Acta Derm Venereol 1999; 79:52–3

26. Haneke E. Bedeutung der Nagelhistologie für die Diagnostik und Therapie der Onychomykosen. Ärztl Kosmetol 1988; 18:248–54

27. Suarez SM, Silvers DN, Scher RK, Pearlstein HH, Auerbach R. Histologic evaluation of nail clippings for diagnosing onychomycosis. Arch Dermatol 1991;127; 1517–19

28. Elewski B. Diagnostic techniques for confirming onychomycosis. J Am Acad Dermatol 1996; 35:S6–S9

29. Lemont H. Pathologic and diagnostic considerations in onychomycosis. J Am Podiatr Med Assoc 1997; 87:498–506

30. Lacour T. The value of histopathology for the diagnosis of onychomycosis. An investigation of 400 consecutive patients. Med Diss, Wuppertal – University of Witten-Herdecke, 1998

31. Machler B, Kirsner R, Elgart G. Routine histologic examination for the diagnosis of onychomycosis: an evaluation of sensitivity and specificity. Cutis 1998; 61:217–19

32. Hay RJ, Baran R, Haneke E. Fungal (onychomycosis) and other infections involving the nail apparaturs. In Baran R, Dawber RPR, de Berker D, Haneke E, Tosti A, eds. Diseases of the Nails and their Management. Oxford, Blackwell, 2001:129–71

33. Gianni C, Morelli V, Cerri A, Greco C, Rossini P, Guidicci A. Usefulness of histological examination for the diagnosis of onychomycosis. Dermatology 2001; 202:283–8

34. Herbst RA, Brinkmeier T, Frosch PJ. Histologische Diagnose der Onychomykose. J Dtsch Dermatol Ges 2003; 1:177–80

35. Reisberger E, Abels C, Landthaler M, Szeimies RM. Histopathological diagnosis of onychomycosis by periodic acid-Schiff-stained nail clippings. Br J Dermatol 2003; 148:749–54

36. Grover C, Reddy BS, Chaturvedi KU. Onychomycosis and the diagnostic significance of nail biopsy. J Dermatol 2003; 30:116–22

37. Baran R, Hay R, Perrin C. Superficial white onychomycosis revisited. J Eur Acad Dermatol Venereol 2004; 18:569–71

38. Gianni C, Romano C. Clinical and histological aspects of toenail onychomycosis caused by *Aspergillus* spp.: 34 cases treated with weekly intermittent terbinafine. Dermatology 2004; 209:104–10

39. Haneke E. Differential diagnosis of mycotic nail diseases. In Hay JR, ed. Advances in Topical Antifungal Therapy. Berlin, Springer, 1986:94

40. Liu HN, Lee DD, Wong CK. KONCPA: a new method for diagnosing tinea unguium. Dermatology 1993; 187:166–8

41. Lawry M, Haneke E, Storbeck K, Martin S, Zimmer B, Romano P. Methods for diagnosing onychomycosis: a comparative study and review of the literature. Arch Dermatol 2000; 136:1112–26

42. Haneke E. Fungal infections of the nail. Semin Dermatol 1991; 10:41–53

43. Roberts DT, Evans EG. Subungual dermatophytoma complicating dermatophyte onychomycosis. Br J Dermatol 1998; 138:189–90

44. Sokolowska I. Acauliosis unguis. Proc II Symp Med Myc, Poznań, 1967:49–52

45. Piraccini BM, Tosti A. White superficial onychomycosis: epidemiological, clinical, and pathological study of 79 patients. Arch Dermatol 2004; 140:696–701

46. Mondragon G. A method for processing specimens of nails. Dermatopathol Pract Concept 1996; 2:41–2

47. Baran R, Hay RJ, Tosti A, Haneke E. A new classification of onychomycoses. Br J Dermatol 1998; 139:567–71

48. Baran R. Proximal subungual candida onychomycosis. An unusual manifestation of chronic mucocutaneous candidosis. Br J Dermatol 1997; 137:286–8

49. Haneke E. The nails in chronic mucocutaneous candidosis. 15th Ann Meet Soc Cut Ultrastruct Res, Nice, 1988 (abstract)

50. Alkiewicz J, Sowinski W. New symptom of trichophytosis of the nails. Proc II Symp Med Mycol, Poznan, 1967:525–8

51. Achten G, Wanet-Rouard J, Wiame L, van Hoof F. Les onychomcyes à moisissures. Champignons "opportunistes". Dermatologica 1979; 159 Suppl 1:128–40

52. Alkiewicz J. Nail mycosis caused by *Scopulariopsis brevicaulis* – Acauliosis unguis. Przegl Derm 1951; 38:28–36 (in Polish).

53. Piérard GE, Arrese JE, Pierre S et al. Diagnostic microscopique des onychomycoses. Ann Dermatol Venereol 1994; 121:25–9

54. Machouart-Dubach M, Lacroix C, Feuilhade de Chauvin M et al. Rapid discrimination among dermatophytes, *Scytalidium* spp. and other fungi with a PCR-restriction fragment length polymorphism ribotyping method. J Clin Microbiol 2001; 39:685–90

55. Lacroix C, Kac G, Dubertret L, Morel P, Derouin F, Feuilhade de Chauvin M. Scytalidiosis in Paris, France. J Am Acad Dermatol 2003; 48:852–6

56. Yazdanparast A, Jackson CJ, Barton RC, Evans EG. Molecular strain typing of *Trichophyton rubrum* indicates multiple strain involvement in onychomycosis. Br J Dermatol 2003; 148:51–4

57. Menotti J, Machouart M, Benderdouche M et al. Polymerase chain reaction for diagnosis of dermatophyte and *Scytalidium* spp. onychomycosis. Br J Dermatol 2004; 150:518–19

58. Ninet B, Jan I, Bontems O et al. Molecular identification of *Fusarium* species in onychomycoses. Dermatology 2005; 210:21–5.

59. Morel G, Raccurt M. PCR/RT-PCR in situ Light and Electron Microscopy. Boca Raton, CRC Press, 2003

Goals for the treatment of onychomycosis

The desired end points in the treatment of onychomycosis are both a negative mycology and a normal-looking nail. Consequently, the goals are twofold:

1. mycological cure
2. clinical recovery of the nail.

Mycological cure

Eradication of the fungus is confirmed by culture (see p. 53) and KOH examination (see p. 52). In many studies, entry criteria require that all patients have a positive culture and KOH; however, the reproducibility of these assessments and their consistency through the study are poor, for as many as one-third of those with a negative culture may have had false negative results on retesting.[1] Therefore, when sampling for microscopy and culture during treatment, it is quite common that there are discrepancies between KOH and culture results for the following reasons. Since the killing rate of the fungi is far higher than the disappearance of the hyphae at the distal end of the nail plate which is dependent on the nail growth rate, direct microscopy may still be positive when cultures are negative. In addition, standard microscopy cannot distinguish living from dead filaments; therefore, some authors suggest that it cannot be used to measure the response of nails to antifungal drugs.[2] However, it is the only objective meas-

ure of fungal killing and is always used in the assessment of treatment.

Since the goal for the treatment of onychomycosis is complete cure, this should be defined according to two important but sometimes neglected parameters, the linear nail growth and the possible pre-existing condition of the nail plate, discussed further on.

The fingernails grow 0.1 mm daily and the toenails at half to one-third this rate (Figures 6.1 and 6.2) As the rate of linear nail growth decreases by 0.5% per year,[3] elderly patients, who have a relatively slow linear nail growth rate, are therefore particularly susceptible to fungal infection.[4] Nail growth is also affected by other physiological and environmental factors such as gender, right/left-handedness, and environmental temperature as well as by systemic and cutaneous disease.[5]

Patients with distal lateral subungual onychomycosis (DLSO) often have a decreased growth rate of the nail compared with that of controls. Consequently, the growth rate of the nail plate should be considered in the pathogenesis of onychomycosis.[6] Nevertheless, a recent investigation has questioned the relationship between slow linear nail growth rate and onychomycosis.[7] The mean rate of linear nail growth in 30 patients previously affected by

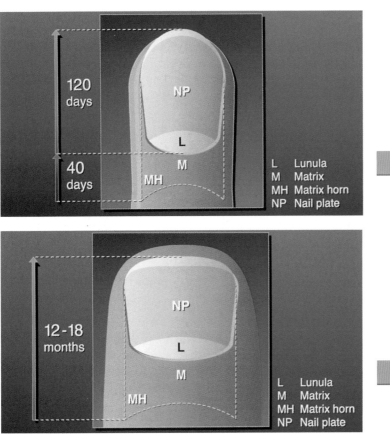

Figure 6.1

Linear nail growth
in fingernails.

Figure 6.2

Linear nail growth
in toenails.

onychomycosis was not significantly different to that of the control patients. Therefore, this study did not support the view that slow growth of the nail was a predisposing cause for fungal nail disease. Other factors such as local abnormality of the nails, which are more common in older patients, may be responsible for the increased incidence of onychomycosis in this group.[8] However, irrespective of the predisposing factors for onychomycosis, it may be tempting to use antifungals (or other drugs) likely to increase the rate of the linear nail growth, since the rapid achievement of a normal nail plate is desirable.

Clearance of the nail plate

Clearance of the nail plate is defined either by:

a) **clinical cure** with 100% clearance of signs, or
b) **clinical success**, with a residual affected nail area smaller than 10%. This corresponds to residual onychomycosis but might include previous nail dystrophy of unknown aetiology.

Chronic trauma implies repeated minor injury often unnoticed by the patient. A history of nail trauma as a cause of nail dystrophy can therefore be difficult to elicit and can be an aggravating factor in treatment. Repeated microtrauma to the toenail would be of little importance were it not for the shoes of the fashion-conscious woman and its significance for the sports enthusiast and in the elderly where impaired ambulation may play a prominent role.[9]

Repeated microtrauma is thought to play a major role in eliciting fungal invasion, especially mould onychomycosis. It also produces a wide range of nail abnormalities which will remain after completion of the treatment of onychomycosis despite mycological cure, since the fungal infection has affected a previously damaged nail.

It follows from the statements expressed above about the accuracy of the criteria commonly used to assess recovery after drug therapy, mycological and clinical cure, that although these methods are simple and effective in many instances, those interpreting the results of clinical trials must be aware of these potential pitfalls in assessment of response.

Clinical measurement and assessment of responses

It has been said that 'the methodology' used for the assessment of response is a 'muddle, illogical in almost all its aspects'.[2]

To evaluate the effects of treatment, the junction between normal and diseased nail bed can be marked by cutting a wedge mark on the surface of the nail (Figures 6.3 and 6.4). Followed over timed intervals, this notch moves distally as the nail grows; the junction of infected and uninfected nail bed coincide if the treatment is effective.[10] However, this method may be difficult to carry out accurately in toenails where irregular lacunae within the nail plate due to onychomycosis may remain and delay recovery.

To assess the speed and extent of the response Hay et al.[11] used area instead of length, to calculate a percentage rate of nail restitution. The difficulty with area is that, unlike length, change is non-linear because the proximal nail is variously concealed by the folds and does not correspond to the nail area beneath. This is not solved by measuring changes in the area of involved nail (instead of unaffected nail) since this area can be altered by nail clipping.[2]

Shuster has devised a new method[2] for measuring nail response that is totally independent of degree of involvement of the nail and the rate of nail growth. The principle is as follows: in the common distal onychomycosis, disease grows proximally; if the causal fungi were to die suddenly, the outward movement of disease could be no faster than the growth rate of nail and associated subungual keratin. In this system the measure of therapeutic efficacy is a dimensionless number, the ratio of the actual rate of outward movement of disease to the maximal possible rate which is the underlying rate of outward growth of nail:

$$\frac{\text{disease movement}}{\text{nail growth}}$$

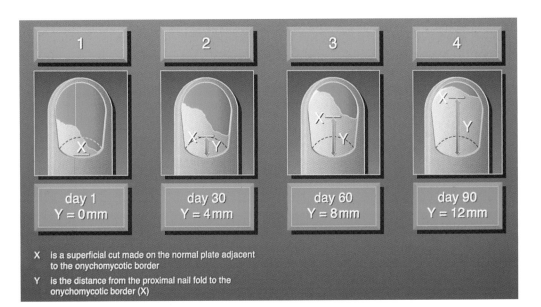

Figure 6.3

Assessment of drug effectiveness.

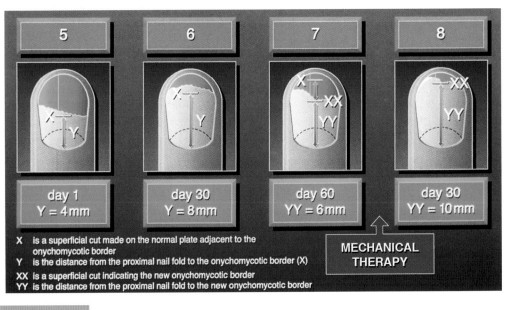

Figure 6.4

Assessment of drug effectiveness. (Modified from Zaias and Drachman. J Am Acad Dermatol 1983; 9:12–19[10] with permission from the American Academy of Dermatology Inc.)

a ratio in mm/mm for length, or mm^2/mm^2 for area.

In fact, the future approach may well be the use of a computerized image analysis system for measurement of areas affected by onychomycosis.[12,13]

References

1. Smith EB. Topical antifungal drugs in the treatment of tinea pedis, tinea cruris, and tinea corporis. J Am Acad Dermatol. 1993; 28:S24–S28

2. Shuster S. Onychomycosis: making sense of the assessment of antifungal drugs. Acta Derm Venereol 1998; 78:1–4

3. Orentreich N, Markofsky J, Volgelman JH. The effect of aging on the rate of linear nail growth. J Invest Dermatol. 1979; 73:126–30

4. English MP, Atkinson R. Onychomycosis in elderly chiropody patients. Br J Dermatol 1974; 91:67–72

5. Dawber RPR, de Berker D, Baran R. Science of the nail apparatus. In Baran R, Dawber RPR, eds. Nail Diseases and their Management. Oxford, Blackwell, 1994: 1–34

6. Na GY, Suh MK, Sung YO et al. A decreased growth rate of the great toenail observed in patients with distal subungual onychomycosis. Ann Dermatol (Kor) 1995; 7:217–21

7. Goulden V, Goodfield MJD. Onychomycosis and linear nail growth. Br J Dermatol 1997; 136:139–40

8. Baran R, Badillet G. Primary onycholysis of the big toenails, a review of 113 cases. Br J Dermatol 1982; 106:529–34

9. Baran R, Dawber RPR, Tosti A, Haneke E. A Text Atlas of Nail Disorders. London, Martin Dunitz, 1996:169–93

10. Zaias N, Drachman D. A method for the determination of drug effectiveness in onychomycosis. J Am Acad Dermatol 1983; 9:912–19

11. Hay RJ, Clayton YM, Moore MK. Comparison of tioconazole 28% nail solution versus base as an adjunct to oral griseofulvin in patients with onychomycosis. Clin Exp Dermatol 1987; 12:175–7

12. Baran R, Sparavigna A, Setaro M, Mailland F. Computerized image analysis of nails affected by fungal infection: evaluation using digital photographs and manually defined areas. J Drugs Dermatol 2004; 3:489–94

13. Gupta AK. Evaluation of methods for assessment of nail involvement with onychomycosis: clinical assessment versus planimetry. J Am Acad Dermatol 2005; 52 Suppl (Poster abstracts) New Orleans, LA, AAD.

Review of antifungal therapy

Topical treatment

Historically, topical nail therapy has met with little success, due in part to the absence of effective topical products. This is regrettable since there are potential candidates for topical therapy such as fungal infections where potent systemic therapy is undesirable because of toxic effects or drug–drug interactions. In addition, some patients may be unable or unwilling to take oral drugs for the many months of therapy required to ensure successful outcome, especially when only few nails are affected. Therefore effective topical therapy directly applied to the nail plate would be an attractive alternative with the additional benefit of a complete absence of systemic side effects and drug–drug interactions. However, many of the conventional formulations of the antifungal agents (powders, solutions, creams, ointments) are not specifically adapted for use in the nails:

- They do not promote diffusion across the nail barrier.
- They are not adapted to take into account the length of treatment required to obtain a healthy nail.
- They do not remain in contact with the site of application for long periods (they are readily removed by rubbing, wiping, washing).
- They are not designed for sustained release of the drug.

Improvement of the conventional formulations led to the development of an alcoholic solution containing 28% tioconazole and undecylenic acid, which has produced moderate results.[1] Penetration of the drug, tioconazole, through the plate is excellent, but is not matched by clinical efficacy.

Transungual drug delivery systems (TUDDS)

A further step forward has been achieved with the development of new vehicles in the form of colourless nail lacquers known from cosmetic formulations. Two compounds, amorolfine and ciclopirox, are currently used in a lacquer base in several countries. These formulations fulfil two essential prerequisites. First, the active ingredient is in contact with the nail for long periods. Second, through evaporation of the solvents, the concentration of the active ingredient in the remaining film reservoir from which the active agent is gradually released increases, thus providing the high concentration gradient essential for maximal penetration. The ciclopirox concentration is 8% in the nail lacquer, increasing to 34.8% (Figure 7.1a). The amorolfine concentration in the film-forming solution is 5%; solvent evaporation leaves a film with a final amorolfine concentration increasing to 27% (Figure 7.1b).

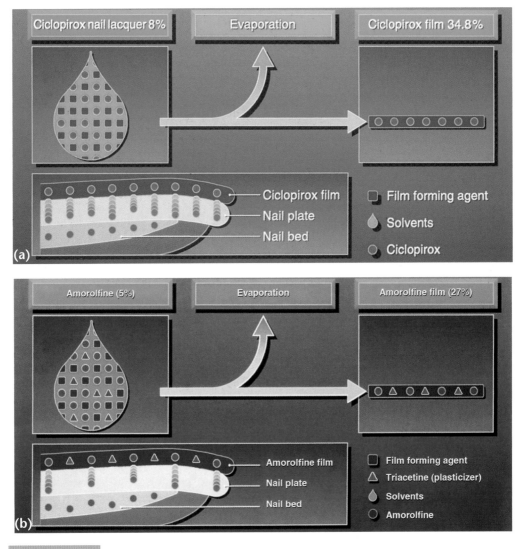

Figure 7.1

(a) Schematic representation of transungual drug delivery system of ciclopirox nail lacquer. (b) Schematic representation of transungual drug delivery system of amorolfine nail lacquer.

Release can be optimized by selecting the components of the lacquer formulation (solvent, polymer, plasticizer) which helps to modulate the release of the drug and maintains the antifungal at a high level in the nail plate.[2]

Because of the additional occluding properties of these formulations, transungual water loss is reduced and thus enhances mass transport of the drug into and through the nail plate. Despite fulfilling all necessary prerequisites, diffusion may be disturbed in nails with fungal channels and splits, particularly at the border between the nail plate and the nail bed. This partially explains why cure is not always achieved.

Ciclopirox

A hydroxy-pyridone derivative is incorporated into a clear nail lacquer containing poly (butyl hydrogen maleate, methoxyethylene) (1:1), ethylacetate and 2-propanol. It penetrates mycotic nail keratin more rapidly than healthy nails.[3,4]

In contrast to most antifungals, it does not interfere with sterol biosynthesis (Figure 7.2a). It acts as a chelating agent and primarily affects iron-dependent mitochondrial enzymes (Figure 7.2b). Consequently, as ciclopirox also impairs transport mechanisms into the fungal cell and in growing cells, there is reduced synthesis of macromolecules such as proteins and nucleic acids.

Efficacy
Ciclopirox exhibits a broad spectrum of activity against several dermatophytes, yeasts and non-dermatophyte moulds, including *Trichophyton rubrum*, *Epidermophyton* spp., *Candida* spp. and *Scopulariopsis brevicaulis*. *In vitro* data suggest that ciclopirox is fungicidal against a series of fungi.

The efficacy of ciclopirox nail lacquer applied once daily for 48 weeks was assessed in the treatment of mild to moderate dermatophyte toenail onychomycosis.

At therapeutically relevant concentrations, the spectrum of activity also covers Gram-positive and Gram-negative bacteria. However, the effectiveness of exclusively topical antimycotic treatment depends on the type of onychomycosis.

Topical monotherapy is suitable for superficial white onychomycosis (SWO) restricted to the dorsum of the nail plate and moderate distal lateral subungual onychomycosis (DLSO). The responses of patients with non-extensive nail disease involving multiple nails are usually not as good. In addition, it is necessary to treat infected skin sites separately.

As the cure rate depends largely upon the severity of nail infection, where more than the distal two-thirds of the nail plate is altered topical monotherapy is generally ineffective.[5] Consequently, when the lunula region is involved or when a risk of failure is likely, combination therapy should be considered as a first step.

Adverse reactions[4–7]
Flares of tinea pedis, skin irritation (erythema) adjacent to the treated nails, or nail bed irritation were reported. These local reactions generally consisted of a

> ▷ Impairment of the activity of mitochondrial haemoproteins
> (catalase, peroxidase, impairment of energy metabolisms)

> ▷ Impairment of the metabolic activities and transport
> mechanisms of the fungal cell
> (phosphatases, reduced uptake of essential substrates)

> ▷ Influence on macromolecule syntheses
> (proteins, nucleic acids)

(a)

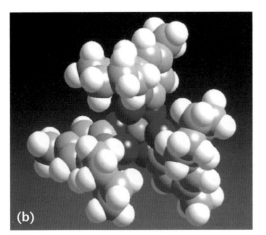

(b)

Figure 7.2

(a) Ciclopirox mode of action.

(b) Ciclopirox–iron (Fe^{3+}) complex.

tingling sensation, pain or intermittent burning and were transient and cleared during therapy without requiring specific treatment.

Clinical studies
In an open multicentre study in 250 practices 5401 nails from 1239 patients were treated with the 8% ciclopirox lacquer formulation applied once daily to the affected nails over a treatment period of up to 6 months (Figure 7.3). The layer of lacquer was removed once weekly. A cure was obtained in more than 50% of cases with a 60% success rate for fingernails.[7]

Two pivotal US studies reported mycologic cure rates of 29% and 36% for patients with mild to moderate toenail onychomycosis treated with ciclopirox nail laquer.[4]

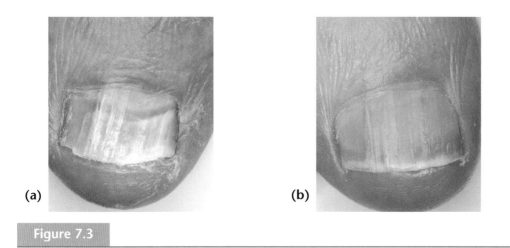

Figure 7.3

(a) Onychomycosis of the great toe sparing lunula before treatment with ciclopirox.

(b) Same patient after treatment with ciclopirox.

It has been shown that under normal circumstances, one or two applications of ciclopirox per week were as efficient as the former daily treatment.[8]

Amorolfine

Amorolfine belongs to a new family of antifungal drugs, the morpholines. Amorolfine inhibits two steps in the pathway of ergosterol biosynthesis, namely the Δ14-reductase and the Δ7,8-isomerase, which play an important role in regulating membrane fluidity (Figure 7.2a). This leads to accumulation of abnormal sterols and inhibits fungal growth.

Amorolfine nail lacquer contains four major ingredients:

1. the active ingredient (amorolfine 5%)
2. methacrylic acid copolymer
3. a plasticizer (triacetine)
4. solvent (ethanol, butylacetate, ethyl acetate).

Efficacy

Amorolfine possesses a broad antimycotic spectrum against fungi pathogenic to plants and humans. Amorolfine is fungicidal against yeasts, *Candida albicans*, *Cryptococcus neoformans*, dimorphic and some dematiaceous fungi, but appears to be less active against *Aspergillus*, *Fusarium* and *Mucor*.

Amorolfine exhibits *in vitro* fungicidal activity which is both concentration- and time-dependent.[9]

Polak,[10] using a microbiological method measuring the presence and the real antifungal activity of a chemical compound, showed that some antifungals are indeed able to overcome air-filled spaces by sublimation, a property of a chemical substance to change the aggregate directly from solid to gaseous without transition through the liquid-phase state. Amorolfine and terbinafine, even at low concentrations, produce inhibition zones over a distance of at least 10 mm through air (Figure 7.4b). The sublimation can be measured by physicochemical methods.

The nail lacquer formulation helps in preventing re-infection from propagules, which are present in shoes, for example. It also helps to increase nail hydration by semi-occlusion, thus limiting the formation and persistence of drug-resistant fungal spores.[10]

For monotherapy, patients should present with clinically evident onychomycosis affecting less than the distal two-thirds of the nail surface.

(a)

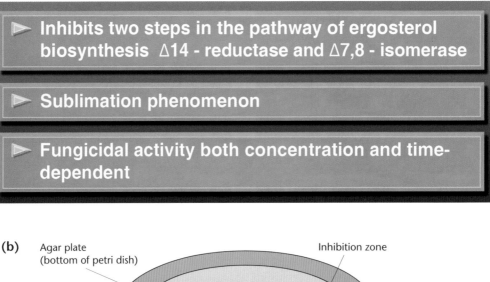

▷ Inhibits two steps in the pathway of ergosterol biosynthesis Δ14 - reductase and Δ7,8 - isomerase

▷ Sublimation phenomenon

▷ Fungicidal activity both concentration and time-dependent

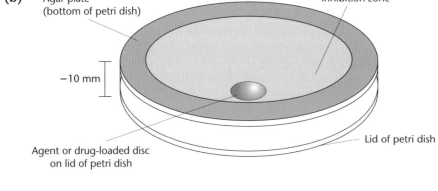

(b)   Agar plate (bottom of petri dish)   Inhibition zone

−10 mm

Agent or drug-loaded disc on lid of petri dish   Lid of petri dish

Figure 7.4

(a) Amorolfine mode of action. (b) Sublimation phenomenon. (Reproduced from Polak et al. Mycoses 2004; 47:184–92[10] with permission from Blackwell Publishing Ltd.)

In the framework of three large studies, 714 patients with onychomycosis without matrix involvement applied amorolfine nail lacquer once weekly for 6 months (Figure 7.5). Mycological cure including negative culture and microscopy was achieved in 52.1% of the toenail mycoses and in 64.3% of the fingernail mycoses. Local adverse events, mostly skin irritation, were reported in six patients (<1%).[11]

Adverse reactions
A bluish or a yellow-brown discoloration has been reported after using amorolfine nail lacquer on a daily basis. Discontinuation of the antifungal agent led to resolution of the chromonychia.[13,14] Reported side effects also include periungual burning sensation, onycholysis and contact dermatitis, as well as two cases of anecdotal painful nail.[15]

Nail avulsion

Filing and trimming of the nail undertaken by the patient are seldom helpful measures for treating subungual onychomycosis. On the other hand, nail debridement or removal of as much diseased nail as possible by a dermatologist or podiatrist is helpful, but only as an adjunct to oral or topical antifungals. It is a logical approach to eradication of the pathogen from lateral nail disease[16] (Figure 7.6) and from onycholytic pockets or canals (Figure 7.7) on the undersurface of the nail, which are sometimes filled with thick keratin and large compact amounts of fungi (dermatophytoma)[17,18] (Figure 7.8). These factors are frequently responsible for the failure of systemic antifungals. In addition, impaired host immune response, inadequate absorption or distribution of the drug and inactivation, interaction or resistance to therapy may

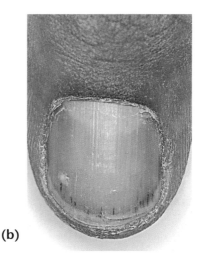

(a)

(b)

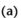

Figure 7.5

(a) Onychomycosis sparing lunula, before treatment with amorolfine. (b) Same patient after treatment with amorolfine.

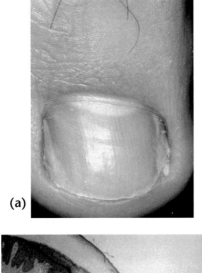

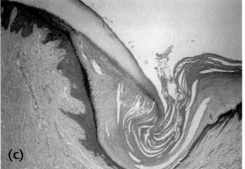

(a)

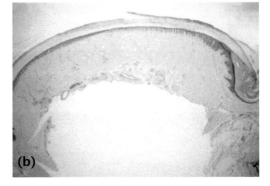

(b)

(c)

Figure 7.6

(a) Lateral nail disease. (b) Transverse section of normal nail unit explaining predictable treatment failure (Image courtesy of G. Rodriguez, Colombia.). (c) Magnification of the previous figure. (Reproduced from Acta Derm Venereol 1996; 783:82–3.[16])

play a part. As in the case of dermatophyte nail infections, nail plate avulsion is also helpful in treating onychomycosis caused by yeasts and non-dermatophyte moulds.[19,20]

It is mandatory to obtain a preoperative history and perform a clinical examination to eliminate contraindications to local anaesthesia and/or nail surgery. Adequate anaesthesia, haemostasis and sterile techniques are prerequisites to surgery.

Total surgical nail avulsion[20]

Total nail avulsion can be carried out using either a distal or a proximal approach. In the usual technique for a distal approach (Figure 7.9) a Freer elevator or a dental spatula is used to detach the nail plate from the tissue to which it adheres, i.e. the proximal nail fold and the nail bed. The operator proceeds by anterior–posterior movements (in order not to injure the longitudinal ridges of the nail bed). The detachment is completed by firmly pushing the instrument in the postero-lateral angles. Then, one of the lateral

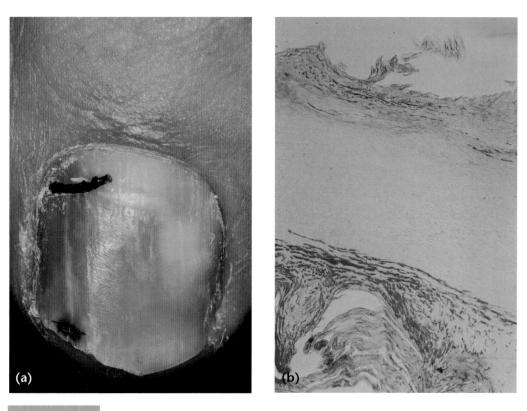

Figure 7.7

(a) DLSO associated with fungal leuconychia as a distal to proximal streak. (b) The same patient, showing histology.

edges is grasped with a sturdy haemostat, in an upwards circular movement to accomplish removal of the nail. The proximal approach (Figure 7.10) for nail avulsion is advised when the subungual distal area adheres strongly to the nail plate and the hyponychium can be injured by introducing the spatula. The proximal nail fold is freed in the usual manner. Then the spatula is used to reflect the proximal nail fold, and is delicately inserted under the base of the nail plate where adherence is weak. The instrument is advanced distally following the natural cleavage plane, and this operation is repeated on the entire width of the subungual region. After freeing the last attachments, the nail plate is pulled out easily. Incidental to removing the nail plate, it is imperative that the nail bed and nail grooves be debrided of subungual debris; this is best accomplished by wiping the nail bed and nail grooves with a gauze wrapped around the end of a mosquito haemostat.

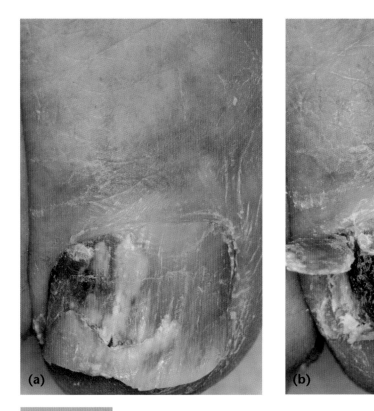

Figure 7.8

(a) Dermatophytoma. (b) Same patient after partial debridement.

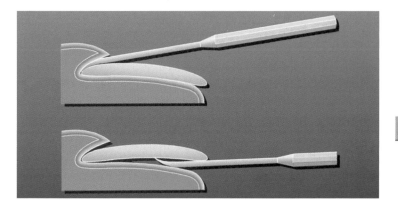

Figure 7.9

Surgical nail
avulsion – distal
approach.

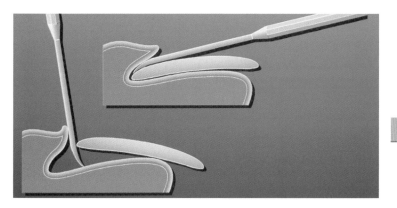

Total surgical removal has to be discouraged: the distal nail bed may shrink and become dislocated dorsally. In addition, the loss of counter pressure produced by the removal of the nail plate allows expansion of the distal soft tissue and the distal edge of the regrowing nail then embeds itself (Figure 7.11). This can be largely overcome by using partial nail avulsion. However, in a small percentage of cases depending on the degree of patient discomfort, for example, when total surgical removal has been decided, the patient should be instructed to use either a preformed plastic nail sold at drugstores and maintained by a sticking plaster[21] or a prosthetic acrylic nail anchored on the regrowing nail plate so that the width of the nail bed is maintained and subsequent ingrowth is avoided.

Partial surgical nail avulsion[21,22]

Partial surgical nail avulsion for onychomycosis can be performed under local anaesthesia in a selected group of patients in whom the fungal infection is of limited extent. It permits the removal of the affected portion of the nail plate in one session, even when the disease has reached the buried region of the nail bed beneath the proximal nail fold.

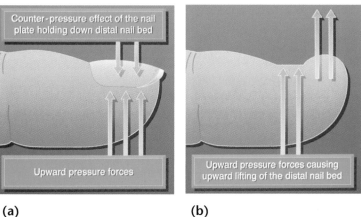

(a) (b)

Figure 7.11

(a, b) Potential risk
of total nail
avulsion.

The diseased nail plate including a margin of normal-appearing nail is cut with an English nail splitter or a double action bone rongeur, then removed with a sturdy forceps as for total avulsion. The digit is bandaged and postoperative care is continued for a few days.

In **DLSO**, surgery consists of removing the lateral or medial segment of the nail plate, especially on the toes (Figure 7.12). Therefore enough normal nail is left to counteract the upward forces exerted on the distal soft tissue when walking and this will prevent the appearance of a distal nail wall.

In *Candida* **onycholysis**, thorough clipping away of as much of the detached nail as possible facilitates the daily application of an antifungal drug until nail growth is achieved (Figure 7.13).

In **proximal subungual onychomycosis**, removal of the non-adherent base of the nail plate is easy (Figures 7.14 and 7.15). The nail plate is detached from the proximal nail fold. The lunula region of the nail is then cut transversally with a nail splitter by inserting the instrument beneath the lateral edge of the nail. Leaving the distal portion of the nail in place decreases discomfort. As for DLSO, in any type of onychomycosis treated surgically, the avulsed segment must always include a margin of normal nail.

Recalcitrant *Candida* paronychia with secondary nail plate invasion is usually an occupational disease (e.g. wet work, hairdressing). It may be treated as a last resort by surgical excision of a crescent of thickened proximal nail fold associated with partial avulsion of the affected portion of the nail keratin[23] (Figure 7.16).

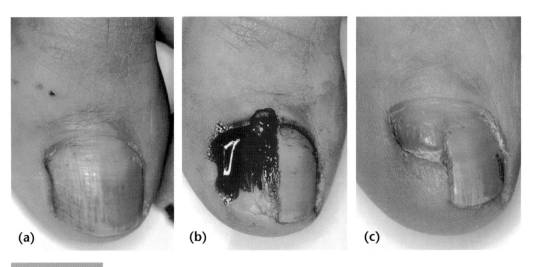

(a) (b) (c)

Figure 7.12

(a) DLSO before treatment. (b) Same patient after partial nail avulsion. (c) Same patient with nail regrowth.

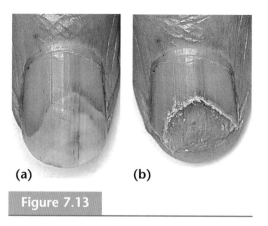

(a)   (b)

Figure 7.13

(a) *Candida* onycholysis – before treatment. (b) Same patient after debridement.

Chemical avulsion

Chemical avulsion is a painless method which has superseded partial surgical avulsion, especially in children and the elderly. It may be repeated as often as necessary. The formulation used is shown in Table 7.1.[24]

Urea ointment is applied to the nail plate after protecting the surrounding skin, for example with adhesive dress-

TABLE 7.1	Urea ointment formulation	
Urea		40%
White beeswax (in paraffin)		5%
Anhydrous lanolin		20%
White petrolatum		25%
Silica gel type H		10%

ing. The entire distal digit is then wrapped for a week (Figure 7.17a–c).

Urea ointment appears to focus its action on the bond between the nail keratin and the diseased nail bed; it spares only the normal nail tissue. Afterwards, blunt dissection using a nail elevator and nail clipper leaves the remaining portion of normal nail plate intact. Following removal of the diseased part of the nail, topical antifungal agents (imidazoles, tolnaftate, haloprogin, ciclopiroxola-mine) should be applied for several months under occlusion, especially if there is no associated systemic therapy. Combination 20% urea and 10% salicylic acid ointment has been suggested.[25]

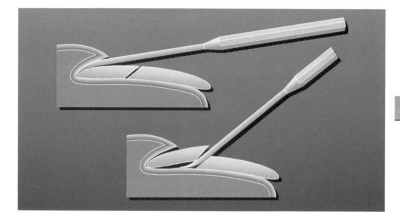

Figure 7.14

Schematic partial surgical nail avulsion in proximal subungual onychomycosis.

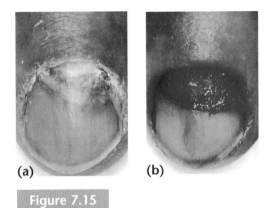

(a)   **(b)**

Figure 7.15

(a) Proximal subungual onychomycosis.
(b) Same patient after removal of the proximal portion of the affected nail.

Some authors prefer to use 50% potassium iodide ointment in anhydrous lanolin plus 0.5% iodochlorhydroxyquine instead of 40% urea for keratinolysis.[26]

A ready-made topical preparation containing 40% urea and 1% bifonazole is available in some countries.[27,28] This preparation is applied under occlusion and the patient is asked to debride the nails every day for 1–2 weeks, facilitating removal of the diseased nail keratin within 1 or 2 weeks of this daily treatment. Then, 1% bifonazole cream is applied once a day for 2 months to the whole nail area and rubbed onto the nail bed. In some clinical trials, the efficacy of this ointment has been demonstrated provided that the instructions are properly followed and that strict compliance by the patient is ensured. However, such treatment is difficult to apply in the elderly, tedious when several digits are affected and/or ineffective when the proximal portion of the nail plate is invaded by fungal organisms beneath the nail fold. Once again, the treatment is more suitable for limited and early nail disease. The unpleasant odour following use of urea ointment, especially when left for 1 week, has led to the development of a new formulation acting as a transungual drug system, which may

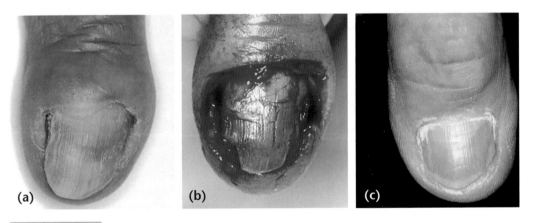

(a)   **(b)**   **(c)**

Figure 7.16

(a) Recalcitrant chronic paronychia. (b) Treatment of recalcitrant chronic paronychia – same patient. (c) Same patient, after treatment of recalcitrant chronic paronychia.

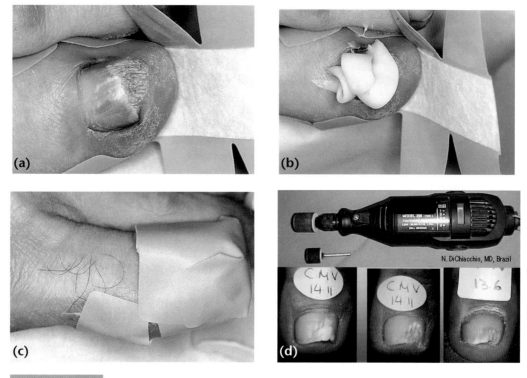

Figure 7.17

(a) Chemical avulsion with urea/bifonazole before treatment of DLSO. (b) Application of the paste. (c) Adhesive dressing protecting the surrounding skin and wrapping the distal digits. (d) Nail abrasion associated with weekly application of amorolfine. (Image courtesy of N. Di Chiacchio, Brazil.)

resolve most of the problems resulting from the chemical keratinolysis.[29]

Nail abrasion

Nail abrasion using sandpaper fraises at the beginning of the treatment with an antifungal nail lacquer, or before weekly application of amorolfine, decreases the critical fungal mass. It aids penetration of a high concentration of the drug into the deepest nail layers[30] (Figure 7.17d).

However, the best instrument and the most useful is the high speed hand-piece (350 000 revs per minute) which can get rid of all the areas affected by fungal infection without any complaint of burning in only one session.

Systemic treatment with new antifungal drugs

The efficacy of the systemically active antifungal drugs – itraconazole, fluconazole and terbinafine – is clear but the frequency and seriousness of side effects should be an integral part of the decision as to the use of a rational treatment.[31] We have therefore extensively reviewed the issue of safety, drug interactions and the spectrum of adverse events.

Itraconazole

Pharmacology (Table 7.2)

Itraconazole is a triazole antifungal agent that is effective against dermatophytes, yeasts and many pathogenic moulds. It is a strong inhibitor of fungal ergosterol biosynthesis, which is crucial for the correct functioning of fungal lipid membranes. It has a high affinity for fungal cytochrome P450 and binds only weakly to mammalian cytochrome P450-linked enzymes. Itraconazole has the broadest *in vitro* action spectrum of all available systemically active antifungal drugs.[32] *In vitro* resistance to itraconazole is rare.

Pharmacokinetics[34–37] (Table 7.3)

Itraconazole is a highly lipophilic substance and well absorbed from the gastrointestinal tract under acid conditions.

It should be given directly after a meal. It is significantly better absorbed when administered in a cyclodextrin formulation, which is used for treatment of oropharyngeal candidosis in severely ill patients. Itraconazole is metabolized in the liver to inactive metabolites 40%.[35]

Itraconazole reaches the skin via passive diffusion from the dermal capillaries, massive excretion with sebum, and incorporation into basal keratinocytes, but little is found in sweat. Epidermis and nail concentrations are much higher than plasma levels. Itraconazole shows very strong binding to keratin. Redistribution of itraconazole from stratum corneum and nail into plasma is negligible. Nails take up and concentrate itraconazole. It can be detected in nail clippings as early as 7 days after the start of treatment (Figure 7.18). Within 1 month, higher concentrations are reached in fingernails than in toenails. Doubling the dose from 100 mg to 200 mg daily increased itraconazole nail concentrations 7–10-fold. High nail levels are maintained for 6–9 months in fingernails and toenails (Figure 7.19). Itraconazole nail concentrations appear to parallel cure rates. The

TABLE 7.2	*In vitro* minimal inhibitory concentration (µg/ml) for dermatophytes cultured from onychomycosis		
ITRACONAZOLE	**FLUCONAZOLE**		**TERBINAFINE**
0.06–0.5	1–64		0.003–0.06
0.1–2	64–1024		0.001–0.05

First line: *T. rubrum, T. mentagrophytes, T. tonsurans, T. violaceum, T. soudanense, M. canis, E. floccosum.*[33]
Second line: *T. rubrum, T. mentagrophytes.*[34]

| TABLE 7.3 | Pharmacology and pharmacokinetic properties of itraconazole, fluconazole and terbinafine | | |

PROPERTIES	ITRACONAZOLE	FLUCONAZOLE	TERBINAFINE
Chemistry	Triazole Lipophilic Highly keratinophilic	bis-Triazole Hydrophilic Keratinophilic	Allylamine Lipophilic Strongly keratinophilic
Pharmacology Mechanism of action	Inhibition of ergosterol synthesis (lanosterol-demethylase)	Inhibition of ergosterol synthesis (lanosterol-demethylase)	Inhibition of ergosterol synthesis (squalene-epoxidase)
Cytochrome p450-dependent	Yes	Yes	No
Effect of human sterol biosynthesis	Weak	Almost none	None
Resistance development	Very rare	Rare	Not reported
Pharmacokinetics Absorption	Requires acid pH	Independent of pH and food intake	Independent of food intake
Peak plasma concentrations	289 ng/ml, 4.7 h after 200 mg	Reached after 3 hours	After 2 hours
Plasma protein binding	>99%	12%	>98%
Metabolism in liver	Extensive	Virtually none	Extensive
Excretion	40% urine, rest with faeces	Completely with urine	80% with urine
Diffusion to skin	Capillary vessels, excretion with sebum, incorporation in basal cells	Capillaries, excretion with sweat, incorporation in basal cells	Capillaries, excretion with sebum, weakly with sweat, incorporation in basal cells
Drug in nails	Concentration and persistence for 6–9 months, concentration in subungual keratoses	Rapid appearance, concentration, persistence for 3–6 months	Rapid appearance, concentration, persistence for 3–6 months

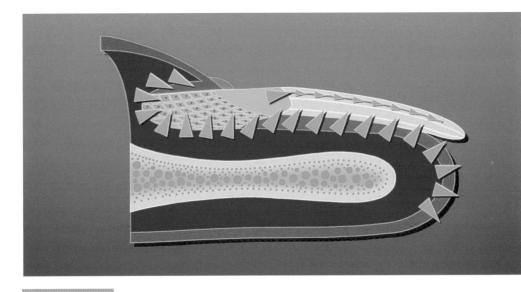

Figure 7.18

Penetration pathways in the nails of the new oral antifungal drugs.

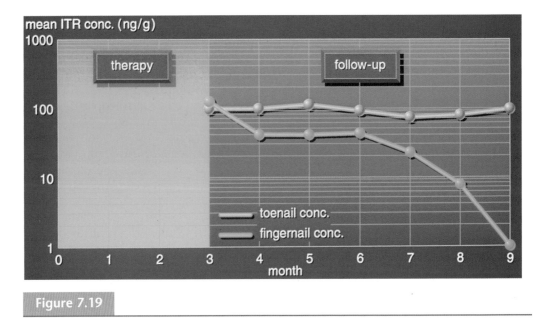

Figure 7.19

New antifungal (Itracanazole) content drugs in the distal nail plate.

drug is also found to be concentrated at the major site of infection, that is in the hyperkeratosis of the nail bed. Nail clippings had 240 ng/g whereas subungual hyperkeratosis showed concentrations of 567 ng/g.[35,36]

Rapid appearance, concentration and persistence of itraconazole in the nail plate were the rationale for the development of intermittent treatment with pulses of itraconazole 200 mg twice daily for 1 week per month, repeated two to three times.[37]

Adverse events and drug interactions
(Tables 7.3–7.5)

Itraconazole also binds to the mammalian CYP450 3A4 system in the liver where the drug is metabolized, although with much less avidity than to fungal cells. This mechanism is responsible for most aspects of potential itraconazole toxicity and clinically relevant drug–drug interactions.

The most common adverse reactions after itraconazole intake are headache and gastrointestinal tract upset. Dermatologic disorders, including Stevens-Johnson syndrome, have been reported. Asymptomatic abnormalities of hepatic function occur in <3% of patients. Reversible hepatobiliary effects are estimated at 1:500 000. Hepatitis occurs most often with continuous therapy, and usually after ≥4 weeks of therapy. Monitoring hepatic enzyme test values is recommended in patients with pre-existing hepatic function abnormalities, those who have experienced liver toxicity with other medications and those receiving continuous itraconazole

for >1 month, or at any time when a patient develops symptoms suggestive of liver dysfunction.

Congestive heart failure and pulmonary oedema have been reported and itraconazole should not be administered in patients with evidence of ventricular dysfunction or a history of congestive heart failure.

Itraconazole inhibits 14-α-demethylase, a fungal P450 enzyme and a member of the same group of enzymes, present in the human liver, which is responsible for the metabolism of many drugs. Itraconazole specifically inhibits the cytochrome P450 3A4 isoenzyme system (CYP3A4), and consequently, may increase plasma concentrations of drugs metabolized by this pathway. Itraconazole is also known to increase the levels of digoxin, certain anticonvulsants, antiarrhythmics, antimycobacterials, antihistamines, antipsychotics, benzodiazepines, calcium channel blockers, gastric acid suppressors/neutralizers, gastrointestinal motility agents, HMG-CoA-reductase inhibitors, protease inhibitors, polyenes, oral hypoglycaemic agents, antineoplastic agents and immunosuppressants. Itraconazole can lead to a reduction in sildenafil clearance when co-administered. Cisapride, terfenadine, quinidine, dofetilide, oral midazolam, pimozide, triazolam and HMG-CoA-reductase inhibitors metabolized by CYP3A4, such as lovastatin and simvastatin, are contraindicated with itraconazole. Because itraconazole is itself metabolized by CYP3A4, any inducers or inhibitors may respectively decrease or elevate itraconazole levels. Absorption of itraconazole may be decreased by the concomitant admin-

TABLE 7.4	Selected drugs that are predicted to alter the plasma concentration of itraconazole or have their plasma concentration altered by itraconazole

DRUG PLASMA CONCENTRATION INCREASED BY ITRACONAZOLE

Antiarrhythmics	Digoxin, dofetilide, quinidine, disopyramide
Anticonvulsants	Carbamazepine
Antimycobacterials	Rifabutin
Antineoplastics	Busulfan, docetaxel, vinca alkaloids
Antipsychotics	Pimozide
Benzodiazepines	Alprazolam, diazepam, midazolam, triazolam
Calcium channel blockers	Dihydropyridines, verapamil
Gastrointestinal motility agents	Cisapride
HMG-CoA-reductase inhibitors	Atorvastatin, cerivastatin, lovastatin, simvastatin
Immunosuppressants	Cyclosporine, tacrolimus, sirolimus
Oral hypoglycaemics	Oral hypoglycaemics
Protease inhibitors	Indinavir, ritonavir, saquinavir
Other	Levacetylmethadol (levomethadyl), ergot alkaloids, halofantrine, alfentanil buspirone, methylprednisolone, budesonide, dexamethasone, trimetrexate, warfarin, cilostazol, eletriptan

DECREASED PLASMA CONCENTRATION OF ITRACONAZOLE

Anticonvulsants	Carbamazepine, phenobarbital, phenytoin
Antimycobacterials	Isoniazid, rifabutin, rifampin
Gastric acid suppressors/ neutralizers	Antacids, H_2-receptor antagonists, proton pump inhibitors
Non-nucleoside reverse transcriptase inhibitors	Nevirapine

INCREASED PLASMA CONCENTRATION OF ITRACONAZOLE

Macrolide antibiotics	Clarithromycin, erythromycin
Protease inhibitors	Indinavir, ritonavir

TABLE 7.5	Potentially dangerous or life-threatening drug interactions with itraconazole
Abnormal heartbeats could result	Quinidine (such as Cardioquin®, Quinaglute®, Quinidex®) Dofetilide (such as Tikosyn™) Cisapride (such as Propulsid®) Pimozide (such as Orap®) Levacetylmethadol (such as Orlaam®)
Patients taking any of the following medicines	Lovastatin (such as Mevacor®, Advicor®, Altocor™) Simvastatin (such as Zocor®) Triazolam (such as Halcion®) Midazolam (such as Versed®) Ergot alkaloids (such as Migranal®, Ergonovine®, Cafergot®, Methergine®)

This list is not all-inclusive.

istration of antacids, H_2-blockers and proton pump inhibitors.

Precautions

Due to its interaction with many other drugs metabolized by cytochrome P450-linked enzymes itraconazole should be used cautiously in elderly patients who are often on multidrug therapy.

Itraconazole rarely causes hepatic reactions. A baseline liver function test is recommended in patients with a history of liver disease, potentially hepatotoxic drugs and excessive alcohol consumption.

Itraconazole dosing

Itraconazole is given either as a 200 mg dose once daily[38] for 3 months or, preferably, as a pulse therapy with intermittent dosing of 200 mg itraconazole twice daily for 1 week each month over a period of 2 months for fingernail and 3 months for toenail fungal infections.

Itraconazole in onychomycosis
(Figure 7.20)

As itraconazole is rapidly distributed to the nails, accumulated, concentrated and retained in the nails for many months, intermittent treatment using a dose of 200 mg twice daily over 1 week per month was instituted, giving the same good results while reducing the amount of drug given as well as the drug cost by 50%.[39] Intermittent treatment is well tolerated, safe, as effective as continuous therapy with 200 mg daily and less expensive.[40] Relapse rates are at least 10%. In a multicentre, double-blind study, patients were randomly allocated to receive either continuous (200 mg/day) or pulse therapy (400 mg/day for week 1 of each month) with itraconazole for 3 months.[41] After the follow-up period, clinical response rates (global evaluation of cured or markedly improved) were statistically different, reaching 69% and 81% in the continuous and pulse group, respectively. The

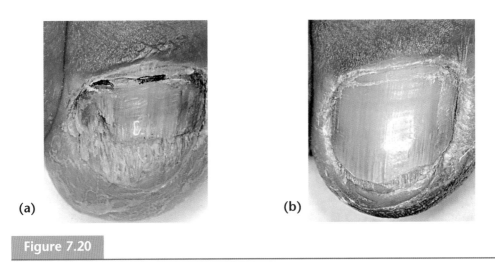

(a)   **(b)**

Figure 7.20

(a) Onychomycosis before treatment with itraconazole. (b) Same patient after treatment.

mycological cure rates for the continuous (66%) and pulse (69%) regimens at month 12 were not statistically different. A combination of itraconazole with ciclopirox nail lacquer in very severe cases clearly surpassed the results of systemic monotherapy.[42]

Fluconazole

Pharmacology (Table 7.2)

Fluconazole is a bis-triazole antifungal agent that is effective against systemic and superficial mycoses. It is an inhibitor of fungal lanosterol 14Δ-demethylase, which is a cytochrome P450-dependent enzyme.[43] Fluconazole has particularly been used to treat yeast infections but is also very active against dermatophyte infections.[44] However, its *in vitro* activity is relatively low and *in vitro* tests do not reliably predict the clinical value of fluconazole for dermatophyte infections. It can inhibit germ-tube formation of *C. albicans* spores in remarkably low concentrations (E. Haneke, unpublished

observations). Its efficacy depends on the daily dose, on corresponding plasma and tissue levels, the susceptibility of the fungi and, above all, on the immune competence of the patient.

Resistance to fluconazole has been observed,[45] mainly in AIDS patients.[46] The mechanism may be reduced azole uptake which appears to be fluconazole-specific, or through an increased fungal cytochrome P450 level which counteracts the effect of all azole antifungals. Other mechanisms include increased efflux of drug from the cell or altered cell membrane biosynthesis.

Pharmacokinetics[47,48] (Table 7.3)

Fluconazole is a hydrophilic and relatively keratinophilic substance (Table 7.2). Its bioavailability is over 90% and it is neither dependent on gastric pH nor the presence of food, antacids, or histamine H_2-receptor antagonists. It reaches the stratum corneum and the nails by diffusion from dermal vessels. It is excreted with sweat, but is virtually absent from sebum. It is retained and concentrated in stratum corneum[49] and nails.[50] It is eliminated two to three times more slowly from stratum corneum than from plasma. Higher levels are reached in healthy nails than in fungus-infected nails and these remain detectable for 3–6 months after the end of treatment.[51]

The concentrations reached are well above the MICs of most dermatophytes.

Fluconazole undergoes extensive tubular reabsorption and consequently has a long elimination half-life, permitting once-daily dosing.

In children fluconazole appears to have a shorter plasma half-life and a larger volume of distribution compared with adult patients.[46]

Adverse events and drug interactions
(Tables 7.3 and 7.6)

Much attention has been paid to potential adverse events and drug interactions related to the intake of antifungals. Before initiating therapy with fluconazole, a detailed drug history should be obtained. The more common adverse events are headache, gastrointestinal symptoms and rash.

In humans, fluconazole inhibits both CYP3A4 and CYP2C9 in a dose-dependent manner, and consequently may increase plasma concentrations of drugs metabolized by these pathways. Therefore, a number of drugs that are metabolized by CYP3A4 or CYP2C9 are contraindicated or require close moni-

toring. Co-administration of terfenadine or cisapride with fluconazole is contraindicated.

Fluconazole in onychomycosis

Fluconazole has been shown to be retained and concentrated in keratinous structures,[48] which is the rationale for intermittent dosing. It is given once a week. Because of its rapid penetration into the nail a 1-day administration per week is sufficient. It was shown that fluconazole was present in cured nails in high concentrations 3 and 6 months after the end of treatment and the concentrations were higher than those of itraconazole and terbinafine.[49] Several studies[52–54] have shown promising results using 150 mg orally once weekly over 6–12 months for toenails, but 300 mg once weekly for 6 months is required for better results. However, a traditional regimen of 100 mg/day for 6 months gave a success rate of 80%, and a similar dose given every other day was also successful, even in patients who either did not respond to, or did not tolerate griseofulvin.

Fluconazole has also been combined with nail removal using urea.[55]

Terbinafine

Pharmacology (Table 7.2)

Terbinafine is the first orally active allylamine antifungal. It is a specific inhibitor of fungal squalene epoxidase, which blocks ergosterol synthesis that is necessary for the integrity of the fungal cell membrane.[56] *In vitro* terbinafine is fungicidal against dermatophytes. Its activity against *Candida*

TABLE 7.6	Drug interactions with the antifungal drugs

FLUCONAZOLE	TERBINAFINE
Drugs increasing levels of antimycotic	Cimetidine
Hydrochlorothiazide	
? Other thiazide diuretics	
Oral hypoglycaemics	
Drugs decreasing levels of antimycotic	Rifampicin
Rifampicin	
Drugs whose activity or levels may be increased	
Astemizole	
Cisapride	
Cyclosporin A*	
H_1-antagonists*	
Midazolam*	
Nortriptylin	
Phenytoin*	
Rifabutin*	
Tacrolimus	
Terfenadine	
Theophylline	
Triazolam*	
Warfarin*	
Zidovudine	

*Drug interactions are usually less severe with fluconazole than with itraconazole.

appears to be species-dependent with fungicidal action against *C. parapsilosis,* but it is fungistatic against *C. albicans.* It is also fungicidal against some non-dermatophyte moulds such as *Aspergillus fumigatus* and *Scopulariopsis brevicaulis.*[57]

Pharmacokinetics (Table 7.3)

Terbinafine is well absorbed from the gastrointestinal tract. Its bioavailability is usually over 70%.[57] Terbinafine is highly lipophilic, strongly bound to plasma proteins in a non-specific manner, and keratinophilic. It is accumulated in the adipose tissue, giving a depot effect and slow elimination from the body. Terbinafine appears in the horny layer within 24 hours after the first dose, attaining therapeutically active concentrations in skin, nails, hair and sebum. Terbinafine reaches the nail (Figure 7.18) via nail bed and matrix by diffusion and via the matrix by incorporation into the growing onychocytes.[58] After 7 days, drug concentrations were 0.43 µg/g in peripheral nail clippings, exceeding minimal inhibitory concentrations of most dermatophytes 10–100 times.[59] Terbinafine is slowly eliminated from nails after discontinuation of treatment. Almost half of the drug concentration is still retained for 90 days at levels higher than the MIC values of most nail pathogens by a factor of 5–50 times. The long-term accumulation of terbinafine enables a relatively short period of treatment for eradication of fungal nail infections.

Terbinafine half-life is increased in hepatic or renal insufficiency.[57]

Adverse events and drug interactions
(Tables 7.6 and 7.7)

The safety profile of terbinafine has been established through a large post-marketing survey including 25 844 patients from 4 countries.[60]

The study was designed with a statistical power to detect rare adverse events occurring in 4 per 100 000 patients. The most common adverse events involved the gastrointestinal system in 4.9% of patients and were usually believed to be related to the drug as diarrhoea, dyspepsia, abdominal pain, nausea, flatulence. In 1.4% of patients they were present as rash, pruritus, urticaria, eczema and headache. In US clinical trials, asymptomatic liver enzyme abnormalities have occurred in 3.3% of patients receiving terbinafine versus 1.4% of patients receiving placebo. Signs of hepatobiliary dysfunction were seen in 1:45 000. Hepatitis may appear without pre-existing liver disease. A cohort study in 69 830 patients who had received antifungal therapy found that the risk of

acute liver injury was increased markedly (228-fold) with the use of ketoconazole, less with itraconazole (10-fold) and slighter (4-fold) with terbinafine.[61] In 0.7% of patients perversion of taste (0.4%) and loss of taste (0.3%) were reported.[62]

Serious side effects are infrequent, but may be life-threatening. Decreased numbers of blood cells and agranulocytosis are rare, as is terbinafine-induced hepatic disease.[63] Marked adverse effects affecting the skin include acute generalized exanthematous pustulosis, severe erythema multiforme, Stevens-Johnson syndrome and toxic epidermal necrolysis and lupus erythematosus.[64,65] For patients with onychomycosis, the German medical profession drug advisory board recommends first considering topical treatment, and prescribing oral terbinafine only after a very careful risk-benefit evaluation.[66] However, other professional society guidelines offer different advice, with terbinafine listed as the first line agent. In summary, terbinafine is rarely associated with certain serious adverse events and patients should be provided with this information.

Terbinafine is metabolized by cytochrome P450 enzymes and plasma clearance of terbinafine is increased by the P450-inducer, rifampin, and decreased by the P450-inhibitor cimetidine.[67] Terbinafine is also reported to decrease cyclosporine levels by increasing cyclosporine clearance. It was recently shown that terbinafine inhibits CYP2D6, a cytochrome P450 isoenzyme which metabolizes tricyclic antidepressants and other psychotropic drugs. Other drugs

TABLE 7.7	Adverse events		
EVENTS	**ITRACONAZOLE**	**FLUCONAZOLE**	**TERBINAFINE**
Overall incidence	10–15%	10–15%	10–15%
Gastrointestinal	Nausea, vomiting, abdominal pain, diarrhoea, asymptomatic increase of liver enzymes	Nausea, vomiting, abdominal pain, diarrhoea, asymptomatic increase of liver enzymes	Nausea, abdominal pain, diarrhoea, sickness, taste alterations (<1%), hepatitis (rare)
Skin	Rash, oedema, urticaria, generalized pustulosis	Rash, Stevens-Johnson syndrome, TEN, fixed drug eruption	Rash, urticaria, angio-oedema, eczema, erythroderma, Stevens-Johnson syndrome, TEN, generalized pustulosis
CNS	Headache, dizziness	Headache, seizure	Headache, dizziness,
Other	Hypokalaemia, thrombocytopenia plus leukopenia, drug interactions	Agranulocytosis, thrombocytopenia, adrenal insufficiency, congenital anomalies	Agranulocytosis, neutropenia, rarely arthralgia, myalgia

This list is not all-inclusive. CNS, central nervous system; TEN, toxic epidermal necrolysis.

predominantly metabolized by this enzyme include beta-blockers, selective serotonin re-uptake inhibitors and monoamine oxidase inhibitors type B. In a postmarketing surveillance study of patients on terbinafine, no adverse drug interactions with CYP2D6 substrates were reported. However, there have been two reports of nortriptyline intoxication induced by terbinafine.

Precautions

Although routine laboratory monitoring is probably not necessary in patients without a history of liver disease and haematological disorders, it is nevertheless wise to have a baseline liver function test and blood count in patients at risk, especially when there is a history of hepatitis, heavy drinking, blood dyscrasias, etc. The safety of terbinafine used at a daily dose higher than 250 mg is unknown.

Terbinafine dosing

Terbinafine is usually approved in onychomycosis with a daily dose of 250 mg per day in adults. A treatment duration of 6 weeks is deemed sufficient for fingernail (Figure 7.21) and 12 weeks for toenail fungal infections. In some countries, depending on the severity of the onychomycosis, the treatment duration can be extended to 24 weeks.

Due to the persistence of the drug for 3–6 months after the end of therapy (Figure 7.19), prolongation of terbinafine treatment duration from 3 to 6 months did not improve the mycological cure rate and clinical cure rates[68] despite some reports not always convincing. The LION study group showed that terbinafine provided superior long-term mycological and clinical efficacy and lower rates of recurrence than itraconazole in a 5-year blinded prospective follow-up study.[69]

Several studies have been performed with pulse therapy; however, no conclusion can be drawn due to the very small patient numbers leading to highly underpowered studies.[70]

Although its *in vitro* activity against *Scopulariopsis brevicaulis* is high, its clinical efficacy on onychomycosis due to *Scopulariopsis brevicaulis* is not well established, with only sparse data on the efficacy of terbinafine in onychomycosis due to this mould. Of 22 published cases, 19 were mycologically cured and 18 were completely cured.[71] *Candida parapsilosis* nail infections were effectively treated by Segal et al.,[72] with 250 mg/day for 16 weeks; 18 of 20 patients had mycological cure. In the study by Nolting et al.[73] using 250 mg/day for 48 weeks, 10 of 13 patients were effectively treated, whereas for *C. albicans*, 250 mg/day for 48 weeks produced a mycological cure in 9 of 12

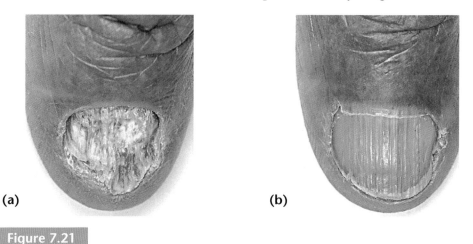

(a)   (b)

Figure 7.21

(a) Onychomycosis due to *Trichophyton rubrum* before treatment with terbinafine. (b) Same patient after treatment.

patients and 6 of 12 were effectively treated. Zaidi et al.[74] used 500 mg for 16 weeks in 20 patients; 33% were completely cured. A longer treatment duration seems to be required for treating non-dermatophytic fungi. Combined treatment using atraumatic removal of the diseased nail plate allows clinicians to use shorter courses of therapy.[75]

Pharmaco-economic aspects of oral onychomycosis treatment

The cost of treatment of onychomycoses is far more than just the cost of the drug. Treatment duration, physician consultations, administrative cost, mycology and laboratory examinations are all factors, and cure, as well as relapse rates are further important aspects. Depending on the method used to calculate cost-benefit, both terbinafine and itraconazole have been suggested to be the most cost-effective systemic drugs.[76] We have shown that a combination of terbinafine with topical application of amorolfine nail lacquer seems to increase the overall cure rate.[77]

Boosted antifungal therapy

The so-called boosted oral antifungal therapy (BOAT)[78] targets resting fungal cells in order to produce sensitive hyphae, which are less refractory to antifungals. This is performed by securing a piece of Sabouraud's agar slide onto the affected nail in combination with intermittent oral intake of itraconazole or fluconazole.[79] The number of nails (9 of 10) cured by itraconazole BOAT was superior to that yielded by the regular itraconazole pulse-dosing regimen (6 of 10).

A similar approach, boosted antifungal topical treatment (BATT), was designed to improve the therapeutic efficacy of amorolfine nail lacquer.[80]

Other antifungals

The last decade has seen the advent of a series of new antifungals which have potential applications for human cutaneous mycoses.[81] However, little information is available about their efficacy in treating onychomycosis.

Other drugs may play a role in systemic treatment of onychomycosis: voriconazole, posaconazole, ravuconazole (Table 7.8),[82] but at this stage there is insufficient clinical evidence. Other substances under consideration include the following: butenafine, ciclopirox nail lacquer in water vehicle, *Citrus sinensis*,[83] eberconazole, *Eugenia cariophyllata* essential oil, eugenol,[84] fluconazole-urea nail lacquer,[85] lanoconazole, micafungin, NND-502, photodynamic therapy of onychomycosis,[86–88] R 1266638, rilopirox, sertaconazole.

A severity index for assessing the response to treatment of onychomycosis is useful when discussing the modalities of its management with the patient (Table 7.9).

Treatment of specific patient groups

Treatment in the elderly

In this type of patient, treatment must be individualized. It will depend on the patient's needs, physical condition, the

TABLE 7.8	Drugs under investigation		
PARAMETER	**VORICONAZOLE**	**POSACONAZOLE**	**RAVUCONAZOLE**[82]
Broad spectrum	Mean MIC yeast 0.82 mg/l	Active against flu-conazole-resistant *Candida*	Including fluconazole-resistant *Candida*
Strengths	Main superficial and deep pathogens	Most deep pathogens including pigmented fungi	Both deep and superficial pathogens
Weaknesses	*Fusarium, Scedosporium,* zygomycetes	Zygomycetes, *Fusarium*	Zygomycetes (NB – *Rhizopus*), *Fusarium*
ADRs	Visual, cardiac	Few known	Unknown

site of the lesions (finger or toes), any associated pathology (which might be multiple), the type of onychomycosis (onychogryphosis, for example) and the possibility of underlying vascular impairment. In elderly patients with trophic disorders of the legs, repeated isolation of *Candida ciferrii* from toenails was recently reported.[89] *Onychocola canadensis*, often involving all the toenails, with a yellowish, slightly hyperkeratotic and markedly friable dystrophy, is probably also underestimated as an agent of onychomycosis in elderly individuals with arteriovenous problems associated with leg ulcers, because of the slow growth of the fungi in culture and the necessity for a subculture for identification.[90] Finally, the clinicopathological spectrum of foot disease may be related to wearing improperly fitting shoes.

A patient in good health can be treated in the same manner as a young adult (Figures 7.22 and 7.23). Nevertheless the management of fingernail and toenail diseases requires different considerations.

The latter may require less medication but more chiropody. This may involve the abrasion of hyperkeratotic nails by means of a specially designed electric file with, for example, a pear-shaped, carbide bit or better with a high speed hand-piece (350 000 revs per minute).

It might be advisable to refrain from additional systemic treatment in patients who may already be taking several medications. However, if the patient is both insistent and distressed by the disease, one could consider a single weekly dose of fluconazole (300 mg) or terbinafine 250 mg daily for 1 week every month. Otherwise the patients should receive only local treatment such as mechanical intervention or chemical nail avulsion, which carries no risk to the ischaemic toe, associated with antifungal nail lacquers.[91] Both offer an improvement in terms of patient compliance and better results as both approaches involve the assistance of a third person to apply the treatment properly.

TABLE 7.9	A severity index for assessing the responses to treatment of onychomycosis	
DESCRIPTOR	**SUBDIVISION**	**SCORE THIS PATIENT**
1 Extent of involvement	Distal one-third of nail plate	1
	Distal two-thirds of nail	2
	Proximal nail plate involvement	3
2 Diffuse nail plate thickening	Mild or moderate	1
	Associated with onychogryphosis	3
3 Nail plate thickening associated with the appearance of linear streaks – includes the change confined to the lateral border*	One streak only	2
	Two or more streaks	3
	If the streaks are black do not score but see 7	
4 Onycholysis	Affecting distal two-thirds of nail plate	2
5 Location	Any one of:	
	second to fifth toes or thumb	1
	Great toenail	2
6 Paronychia associated with nail plate disease	With diffuse melanonychia	3
	With melanonychia at the lateral edges of the nail plate	3
7 Melanonychia† (without paronychia)	With one or more longitudinal streaks	3
	Diffusion pigmentation	4
8 Age of patient	Under 7 years	3
	7–25 years	1
	25–60 years	2
	Over 60 years	3

TABLE 7.9	A severity index for assessing the responses to treatment of onychomycosis (cont)	

DESCRIPTOR	SUBDIVISION	SCORE THIS PATIENT
9 Presence of the following predisposing factors	Diabetes mellitus	
	Known severe trauma to affected nail	1
		2
	Immunosuppression (due to therapy, e.g. prednisolone or disease, e.g. AIDS)	4
	Symptomatic peripheral vascular disease	2
10 Causative organism	*Scytalidium* spp.	4
	Other mould fungi	2
	Yeasts	1

* Linear streaks appear as thin longitudinal lines of opacification or discoloration extending down the nail plate. These streaks may involve the lateral edges. If the nail plate is removed in such areas the underlying tissue is soft and spongy.

† Melanonychia is specifically a black discoloration of the nail plate – it does not include brown dyspigmentation.

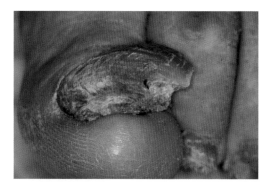

Figure 7.22

Prominent hyperkeratosis in DLSO of elderly.

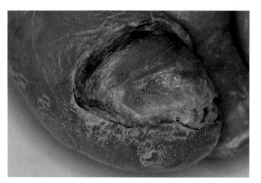

Figure 7.23

DLSO with moderate hyperkeratosis in elderly.

7

Onychomycosis in childhood

The most common pathogen that causes onychomycosis in children is *T. rubrum* (Figures 7.24 and 7.25). Other causative organisms include *T. mentagrophytes* var. *interdigitale*, *Epidermophyton floccosum* and *Candida albicans* in newborns.[92,93] Endonyx onychomycosis caused by *T. soudanense* was reported in two Somali children.[94]

Children with onychomycosis should be examined carefully for concomitant tinea capitis and tinea pedis. Their parents and siblings should also be checked for onychomycosis and tinea pedis. The differential diagnosis of onychomycosis in children includes psoriasis, alopecia areata, eczema and congenital nail dystrophy.

Topical formulations using a transungual antifungal delivery system in mild to moderate cases and bifonazole in a 40% urea cream for thick nails are suitable first therapeutic options. In nonresponders, combination therapy is necessary, as in adults, it will require 6 weeks of continuous terbinafine therapy for the fingernails and 3 months for the toenails. The dose suggested would be 250 mg/day when the weight exceeds 40 kg; 125 mg/day at a weight of 20–40 kg and 62.5 mg daily for children weighing less than 20 kg. In fact, we now prefer Zaias' suggestion of a daily normal dose of terbinafine for 1 week every month.

With itraconazole pulsed therapy (2 weeks over 2 months for fingernails and 3 weeks over 3 months for toenails) the doses suggested would be 200 mg twice daily when the weight exceeds 50 kg; 200 mg/day at a weight of 40–50 kg; 100 mg/day at a weight of 20–40 kg and 5 mg/kg daily for children weighing less than 20 kg. An oral solution is available (3 mg/kg/day).[95]

Intermittent therapy with fluconazole requires a single weekly 3–6 mg/kg dose for 12–16 weeks for fingernails, and 18–26 weeks for the toenails (a suspension is available).

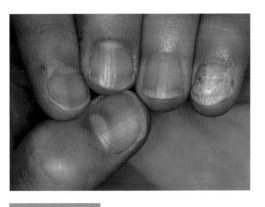

Figure 7.24

DLSO due to *T. rubrum* in an adolescent.

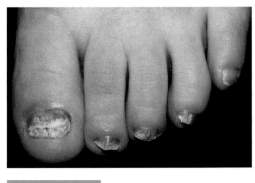

Figure 7.25

Onychomycosis due to *T. rubrum* affecting all the toenails.

Usually SWO responds well to topical therapy, although extensive chronic cases may require systemic treatment.

As none of these antifungals are approved for use in dermatophyte onychomycoses in children, clinical judgement is needed to assess the potential benefits and risks to the patient. In onychomycosis, some advise carrying out blood tests every 4 or 8 weeks, including electrolyte levels (itraconazole, fluconazole), liver function tests (all drugs) and complete blood count with a differential (all drugs).[93]

Treatment in pregnant women

There is only limited experience in the use of itraconazole in pregnancy, but it can penetrate the blood placental barrier. It is excreted with the milk, a fact which has to be considered when treating women who are breast-feeding.

Fluconazole has been associated with congenital anomalies and therefore should not be given to pregnant women. It is also excreted in breast milk.

There is no evidence of an interaction between oral terbinafine and oral contraceptives, and oral terbinafine does not appear to affect the outcome of pregnancy.[96] However, clinical experience with terbinafine during pregnancy is minimal. Due to its lipophilicity, it is excreted in breast-milk and breast-feeding women are therefore advised not to take this drug.

According to FDA (Food and Drug Administration) pregnancy categories, these new systemic antifungal agents have been classified as follows: itraconazole and fluconazole belong to category C and terbinafine to category B. However, it is generally prudent to avoid using any of those drugs in pregnant women.

Treatment in immunocompromised patients

The prevalence of onychomycosis in HIV-positive adults was found to be 23.2%[97] and even up to 30%.[98] A great prevalence was also found in infected children. Patients with HIV infection may be more prone to develop certain cutaneous dermatoses than immunocompetent individuals. The appearance of many fungal diseases in HIV-positive patients is directly correlated with the patient's CD4 count. For instance, onychomycosis is correlated with a CD4 count of 450 cells per mm^3.[98,99]

In AIDS patients, onychomycosis can be observed without evidence of dermatophytosis elsewhere on the skin.[100] Tinea unguium correlates with disease progression. Generalized chronic dermatophytosis has been reported in subjects with CD4 lymphocyte counts of <200 per mm^3.[101]

The same fungal infections commonly seen in the HIV-negative population are also observed among HIV-positive individuals, and the same effective antifungal agents are generally useful, although relapse rates are higher.[102] Besides physical discomfort, fungal nail infection can cause profound emotional distress for patients with HIV and serve as a daily reminder of a disease that might otherwise still be asymptomatic.

Onychomycosis due to dermatophytes is frequent and *T. rubrum* is the most commonly isolated organism, which may even involve periungual tissues. In 1990, PWSO (proximal white subungual onychomycosis) (Figures 7.26 and 7.27) represented 90% of the cases of onychomycosis in AIDS.[103] In 2000, Gupta et al.[97] examined abnormal-appearing nails and mycological evidence of onychomycosis in HIV-positive individuals and noted that the frequency of PWSO in the Canadian and Brazilian samples was 4.2% and 5.0%, respectively. Such a discrepancy in a 10-year interval probably has a twofold explanation: HAART therapy and treatment of oropharyngeal candidosis with fluconazole, a drug that is also effective in dermatophyte onychomycosis.

Gupta's study[97] showed that the prevalence of SWO was 9.5%. Clinically the affected nail appears diffusely opaque and white, a colour which often reaches the base of the nail. It is therefore diffi-cult to discriminate between SWO with deep extension and PWSO that has extended upward. In these cases, *T. rubrum* may even invade the fingernails.

In immunosuppressed patients, onychomycoses due to non-dermatophytes account for only a small proportion of the cases. *Fusarium* spp. may be dangerous in neutropenic patients because the toenail can be a possible portal of entry for systemic infection which can be rapidly fatal despite institution of amphotericin B therapy,[104] which has the highest *in vitro* activity and should be currently considered as the treatment of choice.[105]

Immunocompromised patients present special therapeutic problems ranging from failure to eradicate the organism completely, toxicity and replacement of the most common *Candida* species with others more resistant to treatment such as *Candida glabrata*.[106] The development of yeast resistance in immunocompromised

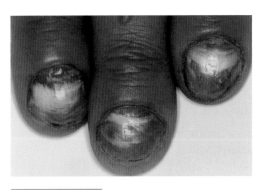

Figure 7.26

Proximal white subungual onychomycosis due to *T. rubrum* involving almost all the digits at the same level in HIV positive individual.

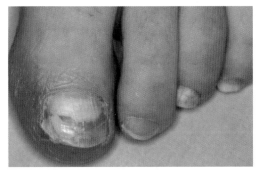

Figure 7.27

Proximal white subungual onychomycosis due to *T. rubrum* in HIV positive patient.

patients is beginning to prove a significant difficulty, especially in AIDS cases.[107] In addition, these patients tend to have more severe disease with frequent recurrences.[108]

SWO due to *Candida* is typical of premature newborns with a transient immunological deficit against the yeast. Chronic mucocutaneous candidosis (CMCC) and other immunodeficiency stages may result in primary total dystrophic onychomycosis (TDO) (see p. 31).

Individuals receiving immunosuppressive medications (e.g. solid organ transplant recipients) have an increased susceptibility to onychomycosis.[109–112]

Rationale for a stepwise approach to therapy (Figure 7.28)

Besides the five main considerations in choosing a drug – efficacy, safety, cost, compliance and availability[113] – choice of treatment depends on many factors including the patient's age and preference, infecting fungus, number of nails affected, degree of nail involvement (mild, moderate to severe disease), whether toenails or fingernails are infected (by which type) (Table 7.9), and when other drugs are taken,[114] special patient population (e.g. immunocompromised), individuals with physical limitations, or with previous failure (not only to topical but also to systemic therapy). In addition, patients likely to fail therapy may be suspected, taking into account some clinical clues.

Patients likely to fail therapy

There are clues to diagnosis and prognosis in nail disease. Removal of an infected piece of nail and scraping the nail bed may afford indications of the possibility of cure, the risk of failure and the identity and vulnerability of any pathogen. A further pointer is that the involvement of the base of the nail plate and decrease in linear nail growth, especially in the elderly, are poor prognostic features for DLSO. Access of the medication to the diseased focus may be critical, due to impairment to the transport

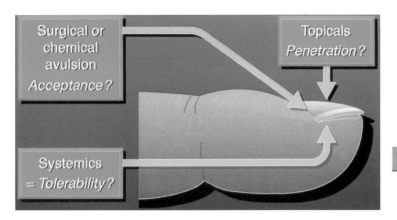

Figure 7.28

Onychomycosis therapeutic options.

of a locally applied drug from nail to nail bed. The newer systemic antifungals may be hampered in their passage from the nail bed to the ventral aspect of the nail plate. In addition, there are four special circumstances where the mycological response is diminished, despite the fact that the drug has permeated the nail keratin via the matrix by the biphasic action of the therapeutic agent:

• Onycholysis (extensive) (Figure 7.29).
• Lateral nail disease (physiological onycholysis)[115] (cf. Figure 7.6a).
• Thickening of nail plate–nail bed, more than 2 mm thickness reduces the ability of drug to diffuse evenly through the affected nail bed and nail plate[116] (Figure 7.23).
• Longitudinal streaking[117] (Figure 3.2f, g), or compact keratin with large amounts of fungi,[118] sometimes called dermatophytoma (Figure 7.8).

More than a need for development of new antifungals, the development of new therapeutic strategies based on already existing medication should sup-

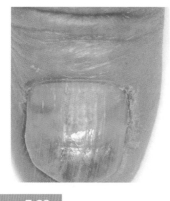

Figure 7.29

Extensive onycholysis.

plement the armamentarium of onychomycosis treatment. Consequently, a rationale for a staged therapy approach in treating onychomycosis is suggested (Figure 7. 30).

Besides monotherapy, tailored therapy is composed of four main strategies that are often associated:

• Combination therapy
• Supplementary therapy
• Intermittent treatment
• Mechanical intervention.

Monotherapy

Early infections with involvement of the distal two-thirds of the nail plate of up to two to three digits may be treated with topical monotherapy using the nail lacquers that act as transungual drug delivery systems. The shorter the length of nail plate invasion, the better the treatment response. Such treatment of distal subungual onychomycosis at the beginning of the fungal invasive process (patients with mild to moderate disease) solves the problem of retaining the active agent in contact with the substrate for long enough to produce the desired antifungal action.

Nevertheless, some patients may prefer to start with oral therapy. The advantages of this treatment are better efficacy and better compliance and they are possibly more economical in widespread disorders and less time-consuming than topical application.[119] However, how often does oral treatment of toenail onychomycosis produce a disease-free nail? According to Epstein[120] this goal is achieved with standard courses of

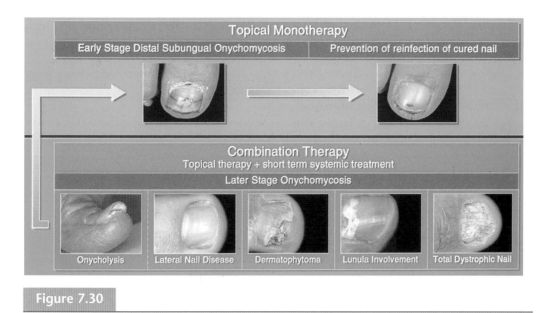

Figure 7.30

Rationale treatment of onychomycosis, indicating which route to follow in different stages.

terbinafine in approximately 35–50% of patients. For itraconazole, the relevant disease-free nail was about 25–40%.

Combination therapy

Since the first detection of synergistic effects of 5-fluorocytosine plus amphotericin B in 1971, combination therapy has been expected to fulfil various hopes.[121]

Oral and topical antifungal combination therapy (Figures 7.31 and 7.32)

In non-responder patients on antifungal nail lacquers after a period of 6 months, one should proceed to the second therapeutic step, a combination of topical and systemic treatment. When the lunula region is involved or when a risk of failure is likely, combination therapy should be considered as a first step and used simultaneously and not sequentially. The nail is then sandwiched between the topical and the systemic routes of drug penetration.

Antifungal combination may increase the magnitude and rate of microbial killing *in vivo*, shorten the total duration of therapy, prevent the emergence of drug resistance, expand the spectrum of activity and decrease drug-related toxicity by using lower doses of antifungals[122–124] (Figure 7.31). Biochemical studies have identified a number of potential targets for antifungal chemotherapy, including cell wall synthesis, membrane sterol biosynthesis (Figure 7.32), nucleic acid synthesis, metabolic

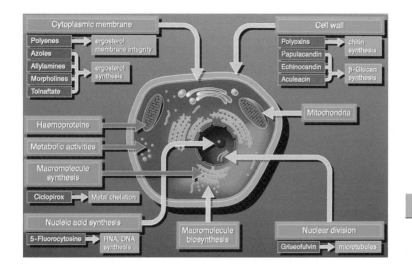

Figure 7.31

Potential targets of antifungal agents.

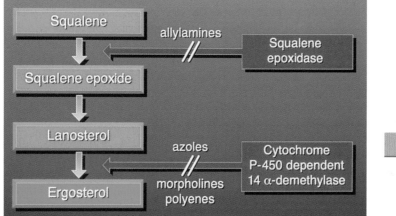

Figure 7.32

Action of antifungals on sterol biosynthesis.

inhibition and macromolecular biosynthesis.[123] The inhibition of cell wall synthesis would, in theory, be highly specific, since only fungal cells build their cell wall with chitin and glucan.

The data from a series of trials suggest that combination therapy using topical antifungal nail formulations and an oral antifungal agent may be more effective than monotherapy for the treatment of onychomycosis. However, most of the information is limited to abstracts in the literature. In addition, some of the studies lack an observation period after the final treatment and a study length of 6 months is not considered sufficiently long to determine whether a patient is cured.

There are two ways to use systemic drugs and antifungal nail lacquer. The combination regimens can be administered sequentially or in parallel. When therapy is sequential, the oral agent alone is administered for a period of time that is then followed by a further period of treatment with the topical agent alone. When treatment is used in parallel, the topical and oral antifungal agents are used simultaneously. Parallel treatment is recommended when patients are likely to fail therapy. Sequential treatment is recommended when patients show a poor response to systemic treatment. A response is considered poor when the microscopy is still positive after 3–6 months of treatment.[125]

Ciclopirox and itraconazole
A study has shown that 41% of patients were cured (clinically and mycologically) and 47% had therapeutic success (negative mycology with incomplete clearance of the nail).[126]

Ciclopirox and terbinafine
In a randomized, evaluator-blinded, multicentre, comparative study, 8 weeks of terbinafine (250 mg/day for 4 weeks on, 4 weeks off) combined with 48 weeks of ciclopirox nail lacquer produced mycological and clinical cure rates equivalent to 12 weeks of terbinafine monotherapy.[127]

Ciclopirox and itraconazole or terbinafine
Medical records of 402 patients with toenail onychomycosis were analysed.[128] A total of 240 patients took terbinafine or itraconazole only and 160 took combined treatment with a systemic antifungal and ciclopirox 8%. Complete cure rate after complete treatment was higher in the combined treatment group (34.6%) than in the oral treatment group (29.08%). The revisiting rate after complete treatment was higher in the combined treatment group (60.5%) than in the oral treatment group (22.2%). In

conclusion, combined therapy increases the cure rate.

Amorolfine and terbinafine
The efficacy of amorolfine combined with oral terbinafine has been investigated in an open, multicentre study on 147 patients with toenail onychomycosis associated with matrix area involvement.[129] Combination therapy is more efficacious than systemic drug alone, faster and better curative effects can be obtained.[130]

Amorolfine and itraconazole
Analysing combination therapy on 78 treated patients, a Korean article considered that it is a promising treatment modality for onychomycosis.[131] The combination cure rate was also considerably higher than the rate observed with itraconazole alone[132] and this was the case in moderate to severe *Candida* fingernail onychomycosis.[133]

Amorolfine and fluconazole
The association of amorolfine and fluconazole is effective and convenient because of its once-weekly application.[134] The MICs were recorded for pathogens that are most frequently responsible for onychomycosis against combinations of several antifungals, namely fluconazole, itraconazole, terbinafine and amorolfine. Amorolfine and fluconazole appeared to result in synergy most often, especially for dermatophytes.[135]

Oral sequential therapy

In a large multicentre study, patients were given two pulses of itraconazole 200 mg b.i.d. for 1 week per month followed by one pulse of terbinafine

250 mg b.i.d. for 1 week. If necessary, a second pulse of terbinafine was administered at month 6 to those patients in whom the response to treatment was poorer than expected. Complete cure was obtained in all 20 patients with fingernail onychomycosis.[136] In toenail onychomycosis, sequential itraconazole and terbinafine pulses compared with terbinafine pulse therapy obtained a complete cure in 39 of 75 (52%) versus 29 of 90 (32.2%) patients.[137]

The sequential therapy regimen was found to have an effectiveness similar to that of continuous terbinafine (250 mg/day for 12 weeks) or itraconazole pulse (200 mg b.i.d. for 1 week a month for three pulses). The adverse effects profile of the sequential therapy protocol is similar to that of the two other regimens. Sequential therapy is cost-effective and reduces the duration for which a patient may need to discontinue a drug that may be contraindicated or known to interact with one of the antifungal agents in question.

Supplementary therapy

Supplementary therapy for onychomycosis of the toes has been considered in patients likely to fail therapy. The rationale suggested by the pharmacokinetic data is that there is a 'window of opportunity' for booster therapy until 6–9 months from the start of treatment.[138] Beyond that point the drug concentrations within the nail may fall to such an extent that a short burst of extra therapy would not be sufficient to effect a cure.

Some investigators suggest that one management approach would be to check mycological status 6 months after the start of systemic therapy, then to repeat treatment for those with positive results with the same antifungal (terbinafine[139,140] or itraconazole[141]), or with fluconazole after a course of terbinafine.[142] For other authorities, mycological cure at 12 and 24 weeks and microscopic examination at 24 weeks can help in early identification of patients failing to respond to conventional oral antifungal treatment.[143]

Intermittent therapy

Intermittent treatment was first proposed with itraconazole using a double daily dose (400 mg) for 1 week monthly for 2 months for fingernails and 3 months for toenails. This technique is sometimes called pulsed therapy. It was also proposed with terbinafine in the same manner or in a different way by Zaias[144] who has suggested a new therapeutic modality for treating DLSO with a normal daily dose: 250 mg for 1 week every month, or 2 months and even 3 months for a long period where the total dose does not exceed a daily treatment with 250 mg for 12 weeks. The only drawback is the long duration of the treatment, which may lead to poor compliance.

Mechanical intervention

Trimming, debridement, nail bed curettage, nail abrasion and even chemical or surgical partial nail avulsion, if feasible, will reduce the fungal burden to a great extent.

The formation of dermatophytoma, sequestrated areas of fungal growth within the nail plate–nail bed prevents penetration of the antifungal agent. Little or no terbinafine was found in the areas affected by the fungus, but adequate levels were found in adjacent unaffected nail. Evidence from this study precludes the majority of the factors explaining failure of therapy, such as poor compliance, failure of gastrointestinal absorption of drugs and drug resistance. These are excluded by the fact that most affected nails have responded in those patients originally suffering from multiple nail infections. There must be a local explanation for treatment failure in the remaining infected nail in these patients. Thus it is unlikely that switching drugs or treating for longer will enhance cure rates. Consequently the formation of sequestrated areas of nail may only be amenable to mechanical intervention (i.e. removal of the diseased material).[145] In addition, oral antifungal may be given for a short time only, for example, terbinafine 250 mg daily for 28 days with excellent results.[146]

The removal of as much diseased nail as possible is therefore the best adjunct we recommend to oral or topical antifungal agents. This combined approach to therapy is a logical way to eradicate the pathogen and to allow re-establishment of effective distribution of the antifungals.

Other therapeutic problems

1) Isolated onycholysis associated with *Candida* spp.
2) Chronic paronychia.
3) Non dermatophyte moulds.

Onycholysis associated with Candida *spp.*[147]

Isolated onycholysis associated with *Candida* spp. often coexists with bacterial infection (*Pseudomonas* or *Proteus*).[148] The nail has to be trimmed back as far as possible (local anaesthesia may be required for anxious patients), the nail bed should be debrided with a piece of gauze wrapped around a stick. A topical traditional antifungal agent must be applied daily. However, unless there is morphological or histological evidence of nail plate invasion, the fungi are generally found colonizing only the ventral nail plate and onycholysis must be managed separately.

Chronic paronychia

The proper treatment of chronic paronychia cannot be generalized since it requires the identification of different aetiological factors responsible for the condition.[147–149] Patients need precise counselling about the environmental hazards that may produce and exacerbate their condition, such as 'wet occupation' (e.g. kitchen work) and microtrauma. Patients with contact chronic paronychia, food hypersensitivity, or *Candida* hypersensitivity greatly improve with the daily application of potent topical steroids. In severe cases intralesional injections or even systemic steroids can be used when several fingers are involved.

If *Candida* is present a topical traditional antifungal should supplement the steroid treatment. Lotions are a preferable therapy, as they penetrate to the site of infection better. Amorolfine has been suggested by some authorities.[150]

Although good responses have been obtained with fluconazole,[151] systemic antifungals are not really useful, except in true *Candida* paronychia infection.

Chronic paronychia can be considered cured only when the cuticle has completely regrown.

In recalcitrant cases of chronic paronychia due to foreign bodies (in hairdressers for example) a crescent of thickened nail fold may be excised under regional block anaesthesia. Complete healing by secondary intention and restoration of the proximal nail fold with adherent cuticle takes place in less than 1 month. As a complement to this excision, the whole length of the affected lateral edges is cut.

Non-dermatophyte moulds

SWO affecting the visible portion of the nail and caused by non-dermatophyte moulds may respond to abrasion of the nail surface followed by topical therapy with the nail lacquers, amorolfine or ciclopirox. Such a treatment should be supplemented in two variants of SWO, of whatever aetiology, by a systemic antifungal:[152] when SWO, starting from beneath the proximal nail fold is due to fungal infection of its ventral aspect and involves both the nail surface and the subungual nail plate, or when SWO that extends beneath the proximal nail fold is associated with deep fungal infection (Figure 7.33).

In the other clinical patterns:

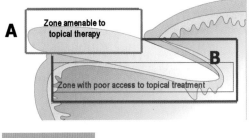

Figure 7.33

Treatment of the three varieties of superficial onychomycosis.

1. Non-dermatophyte moulds are often likely to be contaminating organisms in onychomycosis due to dermatophytes and their treatment does not influence the clinical outcome.[153]
2. DLSO onychomycosis associated with non-dermatophyte moulds only such as *Aspergillus* spp., *Fusarium* spp., *Scytalidium* spp., *Scopulariopsis brevicaulis* and *Alternaria* spp. may respond to intermittent itraconazole therapy[154] or to systemic terbinafine,[155] especially for treating *Aspergillus* spp. (500 mg/day for 1 week each month for 3 months[156]). However, better results can be obtained when systemic antifungals are associated with topical treatment preceded by surgical or chemical nail avulsion.[157] Nevertheless the results of treatment are often poor.
3. PWSO associated with paronychia may result from the same moulds as those observed in DLSO and require polytherapy.[158]

Ingrowing toenails as an adverse consequence of effective treatment of onychomycosis

Approximately 40–50% of patients with onychomycosis have pain. Many have other symptoms, such as discomfort, ingrowing nails, nail thickening, splitting, roughening or secondary bacterial infections; 54% of patients seeking medical attention for onychomycosis have toenail pressure or discomfort and more than one-third experience painful ambulation. In other words, the effects of onychomycosis on the quality of life often drive patients to seek treatment.

However, Arenas et al.[157] reported that 5 of 53 patients treated for onychomycosis (2 with terbinafine, 3 with itraconazole) developed onychocryptosis as a consequence of their treatment. Connelley et al.[159] undertook a chart review of 100 consecutive patients treated for onychomycosis to determine the incidence of onychocryptosis. A total of 37 of these patients developed paronychia. Of these, 19% required surgical procedures to control onychocryptotic symptoms.

Weaver and Jespersen[160] have reported an unusual case of multiple onychocryptosis following treatment of onychomycosis with oral terbinafine. With the new growth of the healthy nail plates the distal aspect of many toenails became ingrown with a periungual inflammation. This required several minor surgical procedures.

Clinically, the therapeutic response is a proximal clearing of the nail plate with resolution of the distal subungual debris.

As the healthy nail plate advances, it may adhere to the nail bed, cutting into the lateral nail folds. This could explain the emergence of onychocryptosis.

In conclusion, clinicians should be aware that onychocryptosis may be a potential complication of effective oral treatment for onychomycosis and the reasons for this.

Recurrence of fungal nail disease, immunological considerations and mycological factors predisposing to chronic *Trichophyton rubrum* infection[161–179]

Information on the recurrence rate is essential for comparison of the efficacy of drugs, particularly for chronic infections such as onychomycosis.

Relapse is simply the re-appearance of the same episode of disease, whatever time has elapsed; re-infection is the re-appearance of a new episode of the same disease caused by a new infection. If a recurrence is the re-appearance of the very same disease by the very same causal organism, this implies that the disease has never completely gone. The somewhat disturbing alternative is a recrudescence from a nest of the original infectious agent that has persisted in the absence of clinical disease – a reservoir rather than an infection, although, pathologically, this is a re-infection, not a relapse. One of the essential pilot studies, therefore, entails careful structural and mycological studies of nails which have apparently been 'cured', to establish whether or not there is persistence of minor pockets of residual disease, or of fungi sequestered without disease. The relative prevalence of these two entities could be critical to the development of a recurrence.

Certain individuals may be prone to develop chronic *T. rubrum* dermatophytosis (autosomal dominant trait); and many infected patients may not be able to elicit a cell-mediated immune response to eliminate the fungal organism. Evaluation of lymphocyte subpopulations and natural killer cells may show that impairment of the patient's cellular immunity is a crucial factor in onychomycosis.[180] It is thought that cell-mediated immunity to *T. rubrum* may be suppressed in chronic infection by a cell wall component of the fungus, and persistent infection may induce immunological unresponsiveness by activating specific suppressor T cells.

Black fungi are responsible for fungal melanonychia. Most, if not all, of the medically important dematiaceous fungi produce dihydroxy-naphthalene (DHN) melanin. This compound is syn-thesized via pentaketide metabolism and deposited in the cell walls of the fungi. By contrast, *T. rubrum nigricans* produces dopamelanin found in the cytoplasm of the arthrospore filaments. Melanins are important in protecting fungi from environmental stress (including drugs) and they clearly enhance the competitive abilities of species in certain environments.[181] The significance of fungal melanonychia is, therefore, that it represents a form of onychomycosis where the organisms are likely to be more resistant to both host and therapeutic mechanisms.

Dermatophytes with high enzymatic activities frequently attack the cytoplasmic keratin of nail cells, thus causing a prompt disintegration of the nail structure. In such cases, an inflammatory reaction in the nail bed occurs readily and is manifested by pronounced hyperkeratosis.[182]

Table 7.10 lists the main causes of failure of onychomycosis treatment.[182,183]

TABLE 7.10   Causes of failure of onychomycosis treatment

1. **Poor compliance**
2. **Misdiagnosis**
   - laboratory tests neglected
   - dual pathology
   - bacterial association
3. **Dietary mistakes** (itraconazole and ketoconazole intake)
   - lower gastric acidity/achlorhydria (for example in AIDS or neutropenia patients) should be compensated by intake with acidic fruit juice
   - empty stomach, since resorption of these drugs (as well as griseofulvin) is influenced by the presence of fat-containing food.
4. **Clinical variants**
   - extensive onycholysis
   - lateral nail fungal infection
   - dermatophytoma
   - paronychia
   - thickened nails
5. **Mycological variants**
   - presence of arthroconidia with thicker cell walls[183]
   - dematiaceous fungi
   - *Trichophyton rubrum (nigricans* or black variety)
   - development of yeast resistance in immunocompromised patients as well as replacement of the most common *Candida* spp. with others more resistant to treatment.[184]
6. **Bioavailability of drug interactions** (see text)
7. **Local predisposing factors**
   - reduced linear nail growth
   - wearing improperly fitted shoes
8. **Systemic factors**
   - peripheral circulation impairment, smoking
   - endocrine diseases (diabetes, Cushing's syndrome)
   - ageing with multiple associated factors
9. **Host response**
   - Endogenous immunologic factors (AIDS, CMCC, chronic dermatophytosis)
   - Exogenous immunologic factors   (immunosuppressive therapy – transplant patients, chemotherapy)

Modified from De Doncker et al.[183]

References

1. Hay RJ, Mackie RM, Clayton YM. Tioconazole nail solution – an open study of its efficacy in onychomycosis. Clin Exp Dermatol 1985; 10:111–15

2. Marty JPL. Amorolfine nail lacquer: a novel formulation. J Eur Acad Dermatol Venereal 1995; 4 Suppl 1:S17–S22

3. Bohn M, Kraemer KT. Dermatopharmacology of ciclopirox nail lacquer topical solution 8% in the treatment of onychomycosis. J. Am Acad Dermatol 2000; 43:S57–S69

4. Gupta AK, Fleckman P, Baran R. Ciclopirox nail lacquer topical solution 8% in the treatment of toenail onychomycosis. J Am Acad Dermatol 2000; 43:S70–S80

5. Effendy I. Therapeutic strategies in onychomycosis. J Eur Acad Dermatol Venereal 1995; 4 Suppl 1:S3–S10

6. Gupta AK, Joseph WS. Ciclopirox 8% nail lacquer in the treatment of onychomycosis of toenails in the United States. J Am Podiatric Med Assoc 2000; 90:495–501

7. Seebacher C, Ulbricht H, Wörz K. Results of a multicentre study with ciclopirox nail lacquer in patients with onychomycosis. Hautnah Myk 1993; 3:80–4

8. Nolting S, Ulbricht H. Untersuchungen zur Applikationsfrequenz von Ciclopirox-lack (8%) bei der Behandlung von Onychomycosen. Jatrox Derma 1997; 11:20–6

9. Polak-Wyss A. Mechanism of action of antifungals and combination therapy. J Eur Acad Dermatol Venereal 1995; 4 Suppl 1:S11–S16

10. Polak A, Jäckel A, Noack A, Kappe R. Agar sublimation test for the in vitro determination of the antifungal activity of morpholine derivatives. Mycoses 2004; 47:184–92

11. Flagothier C, Piérard-Franchimont C, Piérard GE. New insights into the effect of amorolfine nail lacquer. Mycoses 2005; 48:91–4

12. Zaug M. Amorolfine nail lacquer: clinical experience in onychomycosis. J Eur Acad Dermatol Venereal 1995; 4 Suppl 1:523–30.

13. Rigopoulos D, Katsambas A, Antoniou C et al. Discoloration of the nail plate due to the misuse of amorolfine 5% nail lacquer. Acta Derm Venereol 1996; 76:83–4

14. Kim BJ, Ro BI. Hyperpigmentation due to the overuse of amorolfine nail lacquer. Kor J Med Mycol 2002; 7:224–6

15. Lee JH, Roh KY, Park HJ et al. Painful nail due to the use of amorolfine nail lacquer. Third Korea-China Int Conf Dermatol Mycol May 31–June 1, 2001, Seoul, Korea: Poster 51.

16. Baran R, de Donker P. Lateral edge nail involvement indicates poor prognosis for treating onychomycosis with the new systemic antifungals. Acta Derm Venereol 1996; 76:82–3

17. Hay RJ. Chronic dermatophyte infections. In Superficial Fungal Infections. Verbov J, ed. Lancaster, UK, MTP Press, 1986: 23–4

18. Roberts DT, Evans EGV. Subungual dermatophytoma complicating dermatophyte onychomycosis. Br J Dermatol 1998; 138:189–90

19. Baran R, Tosti A, Piraccini BM. Uncommon clinical patterns of Fusarium nail infection: report of three cases. Br J Dermatol 1997; 136:424–7

20. Rollman O, Johansson S. *Hendersonula toruloidea* infection: successful response of onychomycosis to nail avulsion and topical ciclopiroxolamine. Acta Derm Venereol 1987; 67:506–10

21. Dominguez-Cherit J, Teixeira F, Arenas R. Combined surgical and systemic treatment of onychomycosis. Br J Dermatol 1999; 140:778–80

22. Baran R, Hay RJ. Partial surgical avulsion of the nail in onychomycosis. Clin Exp Dermatol 1985; 10:413–18

23. Baran R, Bureau H. Surgical treatment of recalcitrant chronic paronychia of the fingers. J Dermatol Surg Oncol 1981; 7:106–7

24. South DA, Farber EM. Urea ointment in non surgical avulsion of nail dystrophies. Reappraisal. Cutis 1980; 26:609–12

25. Buselmeier T. Combination urea and salicylic acid ointment nail avulsion in non dystrophic nails: follow-up observation. Cutis 1980; 25:397–405

26. Dorn M, Kienitz T, Ryckmanns F. Onychomycosis: experience with non traumatic nail avulsion. Hautarzt 1980; 31:30–4

27. Torres-Rodriguez JM, Madreny N, Nicolas MC. Non-traumatic topical treatment of onychomycosis with urea associated with bifonazole urea in the two-phase treatment of onychomycosis. Mycoses 1991; 34:499–504

28. Bonifaz A, Guzman A, Garcia C et al. Efficacy and safety of bifonazole urea in the two-phase treatment of onychomycosis. Int J Dermatol 1995; 34:500–3

29. Baran R, Coquard F. Combination of fluconazole and urea in a nail lacquer for treating onychomycosis. J Dermatol Treat 2005; 16:52–5

30. Di Chiacchio N, Kadunc BV, De Almeida ART, Madeira CL. Nail abrasion. J Cosm Dermatol 2003; 2:150–2

31. Haneke E. The potential risks of not treating onychomycosis. In: Proceedings of the 2nd International Symposium on Onychomycosis, Florence 1995. Macclesfield, UK: Gardiner-Caldwell Comm Ltd, 1966:12–14

32. Grant SM, Clissold SP. Itraconazole. A review of its pharmacodynamic and pharmacokinetic properties, and therapeutic use in superficial and systemic mycoses. Drugs 1989; 37:310–44

33. Clayton YM. *In vitro* activity of terbinafine. Clin Exp Dermatol 1989; 14:101–3

34. Korting HC, Ollert M, Abeck D, German Collab Dermatophyte Drug Susceptibility Group. Results of a German multicenter study on drug susceptibility of *Trichophyton rubrum* and *Trichophyton mentagrophytes* isolated from tinea unguium. Antimicrob Agents Chemother 1995; 39:1206–8

35. Haria M, Bryson HM, Goa KL. Itraconazole. A reappraisal of its pharmacological properties and therapeutic use in the management of superficial fungal infections. Drugs 1996; 51:585–620

36. De Doncker P. Pharmacokinetics in onychomycosis. In Jacobs PH, Nall L, eds. Fungal Disease. Biology, Immunology, and Diagnosis. New York, M Dekker, 1997:517–43

37. De Doncker P, Decroix J, Piérard GE et al. Antifungal pulse therapy in onychomycosis: a pharmacokinetic and pharmacodynamic investigation of monthly cycles of 1-week pulse with itraconazole. Arch Dermatol 1996; 132:34–41

38. Haneke E, Delescluse J, Plinck EPB, Hay RJ. The use of itraconazole in onychomycosis. Eur J Dermatol 1996; 6:7–10

39. Odom RB, Aly R, Scher RK et al. A multicenter, placebo-controlled, double-blind study of intermittent therapy with itraconazole for the treatment of onychomycosis of the fingernail. J Am Acad Dermatol 1997; 36:231–5

40. van Doorslaer EK, Tormans G, Gupta AK et al. Economic evaluation of antifungal agents in the treatment of toenail onychomycosis in Germany. Dermatology 1996; 193:239–44

41. Havu V, Brandt H, Heikkila H et al. A double-blind, randomized study comparing itraconazole pulse therapy with continuous dosing for the treatment of toenail onychomycosis. Br J Dermatol 1997; 136:230–4

42. Nolting S. Satellite Symposium. Onychomycosis. New approaches in therapy. Proceedings of the 19th World Congress of Dermatology, June 18, 1997, Sydney, Australia.

43. Back DJ, Tjia JF, Abel SM. Azoles, allylamines and drug metabolism. Br J Dermatol 1192; 126 Suppl 39:14–18

44. Fischbein A, Haneke E, Lacner K et al. Comparative evaluation of oral fluconazole and oral ketoconazole in the treatment of fungal infections of the skin. Int J Dermatol 1992; 31 Suppl 2:12–16

45. Rex JH, Rinaldi MG, Pfaller MA. Resistance of *Candida* species to fluconazole. Antimicrob Agents Chemother 1995; 39:1–8

46. Goa KL, Barradell LB. Fluconazole. An update of its pharmacodynamic and pharmacokinetic properties and therapeutic use in major superficial and systemic mycoses in immunocompromised patients. Drugs 1995; 50:658–90

47. Rich P, Scher RK, Breneman D et al. Pharmacokinetics of three doses of once-weekly fluconazole (150, 300, and 450 mg) in distal subungual onychomycosis of the

toenail. J Am Acad Dermatol 1998; 38:S103–S109

48. Savin RC, Drake L, Babel D et al. Pharmacokinetics of three once-weekly dosages of fluconazole (150, 300, or 450 mg) in distal subungual onychomycosis of the fingernail. J Am Acad Dermatol 1998; 38:S110–S116

49. Debruyne D. Clinical pharmacokinetics of fluconazole in superficial and systemic mycoses. Clin Pharmacokinet 1997; 33:52–77

50. Haneke E. Fluconazole levels in human epidermis and blister fluid. Br J Dermatol 1990; 123:273–4

51. Faergemann J, Laufen H. Levels of fluconazole in normal and diseased nails during and after treatment of onychomycoses in toe-nails with fluconazole 150 mg once weekly. Acta Derm Venereol 1996; 76:219–21

52. Scher RK, Breneman D, Rich P et al. Pharmacokinetics and efficacy of once-weekly fluconazole (150, 300 or 450 mg) in distal subungual onychomycosis of the toenail. J Am Acad Dermatol 1998; 38:577–86

53. Drake L, Babel D, Stewart D et al. Once-weekly fluconazole (150, 300 or 450 mg) in the treatment of distal subungual onychomycosis of the fingernail. J Am Acad Dermatol 1998; 38:S87–S94

54. Ling MR, Swinger LJ, Jarratt MT et al. Once-weekly fluconazole (450 mg) for 4, 6, or 9 months of treatment for distal subungual onychomycosis of the toenail. J Am Acad Dermatol 1998; 38:S95–S102

55. Fräki JE, Heikkila HT, Heikkila HT et al. An open-label, noncomparative, multicenter evaluation of fluconazole with or without urea nail pedicure for treatment of onychomycosis. Curr Therap Res 1997; 58:481–91

56. Ryder NS. Terbinafine: mode of action and properties of the squalene epoxidase inhibition. Br J Dermatol 1992; 126:2–7

57. Balfour JA, Faulds D. Terbinafine: a review of its pharmacodynamic and pharmacokinetic properties, and therapeutic potential in superficial mycoses. Drugs 1992; 43:259–84

58. Finlay AJ. Pharmacokinetics of terbinafine in the nail. Br J Dermatol 1992; 126:28–32

59. Faergemann J, Zehender H, Millerioux L. Levels of terbinafine in plasma, stratum corneum, dermis-epidermis (without stratum corneum), sebum, hair and nails during and after 250 mg terbinafine orally once daily for 7 and 14 days. Clin Exp Dermatol 1994; 19:121–6

60. Hall M, Monka C, Krupp P, O'Sullivan D. Safety of oral Terbinafine: results of a postmarketing surveillance study in 25.884 patients. Arch Dermatol 1997; 133:1213–19

61. Garcia Rodriguez LA, Duque A, Castellsague J et al. A cohort study of the risk of acute liver injury among users of ketoconazole and other antifungal drugs. Br J Clin Pharmacol 1999; 48: 847–52

62. Stricker BH, van Riemsdijk MM, Sturkenboom MC, Ottervanger JP. Taste loss to terbinafine: a case-control study of potential risk factors. Br J Clin Pharmacol 1996; 42:313–18

63. Vantaux P, Grasset D, Nougue J, Lagier E, Seigneuric C. Hépatite aiguë en rapport avec la prise de terbinafine. Gastroenterol Clin Biol 1996; 20:402–3

64. Rzany B, Mockenhaupt M, Gehring W, Schöpf E. Stevens-Johnson syndrome after terbinafine therapy. J Am Acad Dermatol 1994; 30:509

65. Carstens J, Wendelboe P, Sogaard H, Thestrup-Pedersen K. Toxic epidermal necrolysis and erythema multiforme following therapy with terbinafine. Acta Dermatol Venereol 1994; 74:391–2

66. Nagelpilzbehandlung mit Terbinafin–Risiko schwerer Hautreaktionen Deutsches Ärzteblatt 1997; 94:B1695

67. Jenssen JC. Pharmacokinetics of lamisil in humans. J Dermatol Treat 1990; Suppl 2:15–18

68. Svejgaard EL, Brandrup F, Kragballe K et al. Oral terbinafine in toenail dermatophytosis. A double-blind, placebo-controlled multi-center study with 12 months' follow-up. Acta Dermatol Venereol 1997; 77:66–9

69. Sigurgeirsson B, Olafsson JH, Steinsson JB et al. Long-term effectiveness of treatment with terbinafine vs itraconazole in onychomycosis: a 5-year blinded prospective

follow-up study. Arch Dermatol 2002; 138:353–7

70. Tosti A, Piraccini BM, Stinchi C, Venturo N, Bardazzi F, Colombo MD. Treatment of dermatophyte nail infections: an open randomized study comparing intermittent terbinafine therapy with continuous terbinafine treatment and intermittent itraconazole therapy. J Am Acad Dermatol 1996; 34:595–600

71. Cribier BJ, Bakshi R. Terbinafine in the treatment of onychomycosis: a review of its efficacy in high-risk populations in patients with nondermatophyte infections. Br J Dermatol 2004; 150:414–20

72. Segal R, Kritzman A, Cividalli L et al. Treatment of *Candida* nail infection with terbinafine. J Am Acad Dermatol 1996; 35:958–61

73. Nolting S, Brautigam M, Weidinger G. Terbinafine in onychomycosis with involvement by non-dermatophytic fungi. Br J Dermatol 1994; 130 Suppl 43:16–21

74. Zaidi Z, Jafri N, Hansan P et al. Open label trial of the efficacy and tolerability of terbinafine 500 mg once daily in the treatment of onychomycosis due to *Candida*. J Pakistan Med Assoc 1996; 46:258–60

75. Goodfield MJD, Evans EGV. Combined treatment with surgery and short duration oral antifungal therapy in patients with limited dermatophyte toenail infection. J Dermatol Treat 2000; 11: 259–62

76. Goodfield MJD, Bosanquet N, Evans EGV et al. Cost effective clinical managment of onychomycosis. Br J Med Econ 1994; 7:15–23

77. Baran R, Kaoukhov A. Topical antifungal drugs for the treatment of onychomycosisi: an overview of current strategies for monotherapy and combination therapy. J Eur Acad Dermatol Venereol 2005; 19:21–9

78. Pierard GE, Pierard-Franchimont C, Arrese JE. The boosted oral antifungal treatment for onychomycosis beyond the regular itraconazole pulse dosing regimen. Dermatology 2000; 200:185–7

79. Goffin V, Arrese JE, Pierard GE. Onychomycoses récalcitrantes et le "low-coast BOAT" au fluconazole. Skin 2002; 5:145–7

80. Pierard GE, Pierard-Franchimont C, Arrese JE. The boosted antifungal topical treatment (BATT) for onychomycosis. Med Mycol 2000; 38:391–2

81. Baran R, Gupta AK, Pierard GE. Pharmacotherapy of onychomycosis. Expert Opin Pharmacother 2005; 6:609–24

82. Gupta AK, Leonardi C, Stoltz RR et al. A phase I/II randomized, double-blind, placebo-controlled, dose-ranging study evaluating the efficacy, safety and pharmacokinetics of ravuconazole in the treatment of onychomycosis. J Eur Acad Dermatol Venereol 2005; 19:437–43

83. Mamta P, Sushil S. Utilization of pericarp of *Citrus sinensis* oil for the development of natural antifungal against nail infection. Curr Sci 2003; 84:1512–15

84. Gayoso CW, Lima EO, Oliveira VT et al. Sensitivity of fungi isolated from onychomycosis to *Eugenia cariophyllata* essential oil and eugenol. Filoterapia 2005; 76:247–9

85. Baran R, Coquard F. Combination of fluconazole and urea in a nail lacquer for treating onychomycosis. J Dermatol Treat 2005; 16:52–5

86. Kamp H, Tietz HJ, Lutz M et al. Antifungal effects of 5-aminolevulinic acid PDT in *Trichophyton rubrum*. Mycoses 2005; 48:101–7

87. Gupta AK. Photodynamic therapy for onychomycosis of fingernails. AAD 61st Meeting, San Francisco, 2003, 440

88. Donnely RF, Carron PA, Lightowler JM, Woolfson AD. Bioadhesive patch-based delivery of 5-aminolevulinic acid to the nail for photodynamic therapy of onychomycosis. J Control Release 2005; 103:381–92

89. de Gentile L, Bouchara JP, Le Clec'h C et al. Prevalence of *Candida ciferrii* in elderly patients with trophic disorders of the legs. Mycopathologia 1995; 131:99–102

90. Contet-Audonneau N, Schmutz JL, Basile AM et al. A new agent of onychomycosis in elderly: *Onychocola canadensis*. Eur J Dermatol 1997; 7:115–17

91. Seebacher C, Ulbricht H, Wörz K. Topical therapy of onychomycoses in geriatric patients. TW Dermatol 1993; 23:434–8

92. Gupta AK, Skinner AR. Onychomycosis in children: a brief overview with treatment strategies. Pediatr Dermatol 2004; 21:74–9

93. Suarez S. New antifungal therapy for children. In James WD, Cockerell J, Dzubow LM et al., eds. Adv Dermatol 1997; 12:195–209

94. Fletcher CL, Moore K, Hay RJ. Endonyx onychomycosis due to *T. soudanense* in two Somalian siblings. Br J Dermatol 2001; 145:687–8

95. Gupta AK, Chang P, del Rosso JQ et al. Onychomycosis in children: prevalence and management. Pediatr Dermatol 1998; 15:464–71

96. Williams TG, Hall M. Lack of interaction of oral terbinafine with oral contraceptives and healthy babies in a postmarketing surveillance study. Fifth Annual International Summit on Cutaneous Antifungal Therapy. Singapore, 1998: abstract 67

97. Gupta AK, Taborda P, Taborda V et al. Epidemiology and prevalence of onychomycosis in HIV-positive individuals. Int J Dermatol 2000; 39:746–53

98. Cribier B, Leiva Mena M, Rey D et al. Nail changes in patients infected with immunodeficiency virus. A prospective controlled study. Arch Dermatol 1998; 134:1216–20

99. Conant MA. The AIDS epidemic. J Am Acad Dermatol 1994; 31:S47–S50

100. Ravnborg L, Baastrup N, Svejgaard E. Onychomycosis in HIV-infected patients. Acta Derm Venereol 1998; 78:151–2

101. Goldman GD, Bolognia JL. HIV-related skin disease: managing fungal infections. J Respir Dis 1997; 18:14–20

102. Herranz P, Garcia J, De Lucas R et al. Toenail onychomycosis in patients with acquired immune deficiency syndrome: treatment with terbinafine. Br J Dermatol 1997; 139:577–80

103. Dompmartin D, Dompmartin A, Deluol AM et al. Onychomycosis and AIDS. Int J Dermatol 1990; 29:337

104. Arrese JE, Piérard-Franchimont C, Piérard GE. Fatal hyalohyphomycosis following *Fusarium* onychomycosis in an immunocompromised patient. Am J Dermatopathol 1996; 18:196–8

105. Martino P, Gastaldi R, Raccah R et al. Clinical patterns of *Fusarium* infections in immunocompromised patients. J Infect 1994; 28 Suppl 1:7–15

106. Evans EGV. Causative pathogens in onychomycosis and the possibility of treatment resistance: a review. J Am Acad Dermatol 1998; 38:S32–S36

107. Roberts DT. Cutaneous candidosis. Dermatol Therapy 1997; 3:26–36

108. Lemak NA, Duvic M. Superficial fungal infections in HIV and AIDS. Dermatol Therapy 1997; 3:84–90

109. Chugh KS, Sharma SC, Singh V et al. Spectrum of dermatological lesions in renal allograft recipient in a tropical environment. Dermatology 1994; 188:108–12

110. Gülec AT, Demirbilek M, Seckin D et al. Superficial fungal infection in 102 renal transplant recipients. A case control. J Am Acad Dermatol 2003; 49:187–92

111. Virgili A, Zampino MR, La Malfa V. Prevalence of superficial dermatomycoses in 73 renal transplant recipients. Dermatology 1999; 199:31–4

112. Weglowska J, Szepietowski J, Walow B et al. Onychomycosis in renal transplant recipient. Part II. Mycological aspects. Mikok Lek 2003; 10:307–11

113. Gupta AK, Scher RK de Doncker P. Current management of onychomycosis. Dermatol Clin 1997; 15:121–35

114. Denning DW, Evans EG, Kibbler CC et al. Fungal nail disease: a guide to good practice. BMJ 1995; 311:1271–81

115. Baran R, De Doncker P. Lateral edge involvement indicates poor prognosis for treating onychomycosis with the new systemic antifungals. Acta Derm Venereol 1996; 73:82–3

116. Sommer S, Sheean-Dare RA, Goodfield MJD, Evans EGV. Prediction of outcome in the treatment of onychomycosis. Clin Exp Dermatol 2003; 28:425–8

117. Hay RJ. Chronic dermatophyte infections. In Verbov J, ed. Superficial Fungal Infections. Lancaster, UK, MTP Press, 1986:23–4

118. Roberts DT, Evans EGV. Subungual dermatophytoma complicating dermatophyte onychomycosis. Br J Dermatol 1998; 138:189–90

119. Frederiksson T. The pros and cons of an oral treatment of dermatomycosis. Dermatologica 1984; 169 Suppl 1:67–8

120. Epstein E. How often does oral treatment of toenail onychomycosis produce a disease-free nail? An analysis of published data. Arch Dermatol 1998; 134:1551–4

121. Polack A. The past, present and future of antimycotic combination therapy. Mycoses 1999; 42:355–70

122. Nolting S. Onychomycosis. New approaches in therapy. Proceedings of the 19th World Congress of Dermatology, Sydney, 1997:12

123. Ghannoum MA. Future of antimycotic therapy. Dermatol Therapy 1997; 3:104–11

124. Polak-Wyss A. Mechanism of action of antifungals and combination therapy. J Eur Acad Dermatol Venereol 1995; 4 Suppl 1:511–16

125. Olafsson J, Sigurgeirsson B, Baran R. Combination therapy for onychomycosis. Br J Dermatol 2003; 149 Suppl 64:15–18

126. Gupta AK, Fleckman P, Baran R. Ciclopirox nail lacquer topical solution 8% in the treatment of toenail onychomycosis. J Am Acad Dermatol 2000; 43:S70–S80

127. Gupta AK and the Onychomycosis Combination Therapy Study Group. Ciclopirox topical solution, 8% combined with oral terbinafine to treat onychomycosis: a randomized, evaluator-blinded study. J Drugs Dermatol 2005; 4:481–5

128. Kim HC, Jung KB, Shin DH et al. Comparison of compliance and cure rate of systemic antifungal therapy versus combination therapy with systemic and topical agent in toenail onychomycosis. Kor J Med Mycol 2002; 7:35–41

129. Baran R, Feuilhade M, Datry A et al. A randomized trial of amorolfine 5% solution nail lacquer combined with oral terbinafine compared with terbinafine alone in the treatment of dermatophytic toenail onychomycosis affecting the nail region. Br J Dermatol 2000; 142:1177

130. Baran E, Bochenski J, Duczkowski M et al. Combination therapy for onychomycosis with amorolfine nail lacquer and oral antifungal agents. Mikol Lek 2003; 10:79–83

131. Yoon YH, An JY, Ro BI. Experience of combination treatment of toenail onychomycosis with oral itraconazole and topical 5% amorolfine nail lacquer. Kor J Med Mycol 2004; 9:159–65

132. Lecha M, Alsina M, Torres M et al. Amorolfine and itraconazole combination for severe toenail onychomycosis: results of an open randomised trial in Spain. Br J Dermatol 2001; 145 Suppl 60: 21–6

133. Rigopoulos D, Katoulis A, Ioannides D et al. A randomised trial of amorolfine 5% solution nail lacquer in association with itraconazole pulse therapy compared with itraconazole alone in the treatment of *Candida* fingernail onychomycosis. Br J Dermatol 2003; 149:151

134. Sergeev Y, Sergeev A. Pulsed combination therapy: the new option for onychomycosis. Mycoses 2001; 44 Suppl 1:68

135. Harman S, Ashbee HR, Evans EG. Testing of antifungal combinations against yeasts and dermatophytes. J Dermatol Treat 2004; 15:104–7

136. Gupta AK, Konnikov N, Lynde CW. Sequential pulse therapy with itraconazole and terbinafine to treat onychomycosis of the fingernails. J Dermatol Treat 2000; 11:151–4

137. Gupta AK, Lyde CW, Konnikov N. Single-blind, randomized, prospective study of sequential itraconazole and terbinafine pulse compared with terbinafine pulse for the treatment of toenail onychomycosis. J Am Acad Dermatol 2001; 44:485–91

138. Gupta AK, Del Rosso JQ. An evaluation of intermittent therapy used to treat onychomycosis and other dermatomycoses with the oral antifungal agents. Int J Dermatol 2000; 39:401–11

139. Tausch I, Bräutigam M, Weiding G. Evaluation of 6 weeks treatment of terbinafine in tinea unguium in a double-blind trial comparing 6 and 12 weeks therapy. Br J Dermatol 1997; 136:737–42

140. Watson A, Marley J, Ellis D et al. Terbinafine in onychomycosis of the toenail: a novel treatment protocol. J Am Acad Dermatol 1995; 33:775–9

141. Haneke E, Ring J, Abeck D. Efficacy of itraconazole pulse treatment in onychomycosis. HGZ Hautkr 1997; 72:737–40

142. De Cuyper C. Therapeutic approach of recalcitrant toenail onychomycosis. Fifth Internatiional Summit on Cutaneous Antifungal Therapy. Singapore, 1998:abstract 26

143. Sigurgeirsson B, Paul C, Curran D, Evans EGV. Prognostic factors of mycological cure following treatment of onychomycosis with oral antifungal agents. Br J Dermatol 2002; 147:1241–3

144. Zaias N, Rebell G. The successful treatment of *Trichophyton rubrum* nail bed (distal subungual) onychomycosis with intermittent pulse-dosed terbinafine. Arch Dermatol 2004; 140:691–5

145. Di Chiacchio N, Kadunc BV, De Almeida ART et al. Nail abrasion. J Cosm Dermatol 2003; 2:150–2

146. Goodfield MJD, Evans EGV. Combined treatment with surgery and short duration oral antifungal therapy in patients with limited dermatophyte toenail infection. J Dermatol Treat 2000; 11:259–62

147. Daniel CR, Daniel MP, Daniel CM et al. Chronic paronychia and onycholysis: a thirteen-year experience. Cutis 1996; 58:397–401

148. Elewski BE. Bacterial infection in a patient with onychomycosis. J Am Acad Dermatol 1997; 37:493–4

149. Tosti A, Piraccini BM. Paronychia. In Amin S, Maibach H, eds. Contact Urticaria Syndrome. Boca Raton, FL, CRS press, 1997:276–8

150. Lestringant GG, Nsanze H, Nada M. Effectiveness of amorolfine 5% nail lacquer in the treatment of long-duration *Candida* onychomycosis with chronic paronychia. J Dermatol Treat 1996; 7:89–92

151. Amichai B, Shiri J. Fluconazole 50 mg/day therapy in the management of chronic paronychia. J Dermatol Treat 1999; 10:199–200

152. Baran R , Hay R, Perrin Ch. Superficial white onychomycosis revisited. J Eur Acad Dermatol Venereol 2004; 18:569–71

153. Ellis DH, Marley JE, Watson AB. Significance of non-dermatophyte moulds and yeasts in onychomycosis. Dermatology 1997; 194 Suppl 1:40–2

154. De Doncker P, Scher RK, Baran R et al. Itraconazole therapy is effective for pedal onychomycosis caused by some non dermatophyte molds and in mixed infection by dermatophytes and molds. A multicenter study with 36 patients. J Am Acad Dermatol 1997; 36:173–7

155. Nolting S, Brautigam M, Weidinger G. Terbinafine in onychomycosis with involvement by non-dermatophytic fungi. Br J Dermatol 1994, 130 Suppl 43:16–21

156. Gianni C, Romano C. Clinical and histological aspects of toenail onychomycosis caused by *Aspergillus* spp.: 34 cases treated with weekly intermittent Terbinafine. Dermatology 2004; 209:104–10

157. Arenas R, Dominguez-Cherit J, Fernandez L. Open randomized comparison of itraconazole versus terbinafine in onychomycosis. Int J Dermatol 1995; 34:138–43

158. Baran R. Nail fungal infections and treatment. Hand Clin 2002; 18:625–8

159. Connelley LK, Dinehart SM, McDonald R. Onychocryptosis associated with the treatment of onychomycosis. J Am Podiatr Med Assoc 1999; 89:424–6

160. Weaver TD, Jespersen DL. Multiple onychocryptosis following treatment of onychomycosis with oral terbinafine. Cutis 2000; 66:211–12

161. Gupta AK, Baran R, Summerbell R. Onychomycosis: strategies to improve efficacy and reduce recurrence. J Eur Acad Dermatol Venereol 2002; 16:579–86

162. Shuster S, Baran R. Recurrence of fungal nail disease and the dissociation of relapse from re-infection. Acta Derm Venereol 2001; 81:154–5

163. Ogawa H, Summerbell RC, Clemons KV et al. Dermatophytes and host defence in cutaneous mycoses. Med Mycol 1998; 36:166–73

164. Woodfolk JA, Platts-Mills TA. The immune response to dermatophytes. Res Immunol 1998; 149:436–45

165. Wagner DK, Sohnle PG. Cutaneous defenses against dermatophytes and yeasts. Clin Microbiol Rev 1995; 8:317–35

166. Jones HE. Cell-mediated immunity in the immunopathogenesis of dermatophytosis. Acta Derm Venereol 1986; Suppl 121:73–83

167. Jones HE. Factors involved in producing a sustained experimental dermatophyte infection (*Trichophyton mentagrophytes*). Cutis 2001; 67:18–19

168. Svejgaard E. Humoral antibody responses in the immunopathogenesis of dermatophytosis. Acta Derm Venereol 1986; 121 Suppl: 85–91

169. Kaaman T. Cell-mediated reactivity in dermatophytosis: differences in skin responses to purified *Trichophyton* in tinea pedis and tinea cruris. Acta Derm Venereol 1981; 61:119–23

170. Dahl MV, Grando SA. Chronic dermatophytosis: what is special about *Trichophyton rubrum*? Adv Dermatol 1994; 9:97–109

171. Dahl MV. Dermatophytosis and the immune response. J Am Acad Dermatol 1994; 31:S34–S41

172. Zaias N, Rebell G. Chronic dermatophytosis caused by *Trichophyton rubrum*. J Am Acad Dermatol 1996; 35:S17–S20

173. Artis WM, Jones HE. The effect of human lymphokine on the growth of *Trichophyton mentagrophytes*. J Invest Dermatol 1982; 74:131–4

174. Poulain D, Tronchin G, Vernes A, Delabre M, Biguet J. Experimental study of resistance to infection by *Trichophyton mentagrophytes*: demonstration of memory skin cells. J Invest Dermatol 1982; 74:205–9

175. Kaaman T. Dermatophyte antigens and cell-mediated immunity in dermatophytosis. Curr Top Med Mycol 1985; 1:117–34

176. Hernandez AD, Reece RE, Zucker AH. *Trichophyton mentagrophytes* spores differ from mycelia in the ability to induce pustules and activate complement. J Invest Dermatol 1986; 87:683–7

177. Ninomiya J, Ide M, Ito Y, Takiuchi I. Experimental penetration of *Trichophyton mentagrophytes* into the human stratum corneum. Mycopathologia 1998; 141:153–7

178. Jones HE. Immune response and host resistance of humans to dermatophyte infection. J Am Acad Dermatol 1993; 28:S12–S18

179. Galitz J, Schein JR. Symptom improvement in patients with onychomycosis receiving oral antifungal therapy. South Med J 2002; 95:1359–60

180. Maleszka R, Adamski Z, Dworacki G. Evaluation of lymphocytic subpopulations and natural killers in peripheral blood of patients treated for dermatophyte onychomycosis. Mycoses 2001; 44:487–92

181. Perrin R, Baran R. Longitudinal melanonychia caused by *Trichophyton rubrum*. J Am Acad Dermatol 1994; 31:311–16

182. Maleszka R. Enzymatic activity of dermatophytes in various forms of onychomycosis. Mikol Lek 1999; 6:77–83

183. De Doncker P, Degreef H, André J, Pierard G. Why are some with onychomycosis still not responding to the newer antifungal agents? Orlando, AAD, 1998:poster 187

184. Roberts DT. Cutaneous candidosis. Dermatol Therapy 1997; 3:26–36

Preventive measures

Despite an excellent therapeutic response to terbinafine (82% clinical cure or with minimal residual lesions as well as 82% mycological cure maintained after 2 years),[1-3] long-term results for some patients with onychomycosis treated with the new systemic antifungals are somewhat disappointing.

A study reported the 3-year follow-up of a group of 47 'cured' patients with toenail onychomycosis using a 4-month course of either terbinafine or itraconazole. The relapses were more common in patients treated with pulsed itraconazole (36.3%) than in patients treated with continuous (16.6%) or intermittent (15.3%) terbinafine.[4] This was confirmed in a double-blind comparative trial of terbinafine 250 mg/day versus itraconazole 200 mg/day for 12 weeks.[5]

In another study of 88 patients, 36 weeks after cessation of 12 weeks of itraconazole (continuous or pulse) therapy, total clinical cure was achieved in 35% of these patients, 93% of whom had negative cultures. At a follow-up at week 104 the total clinical cure was 39%, with negative cultures in 57%. Younger patients showed significantly better clinical cure rates at week 36 than older patients, possibly due to faster nail growth.[6] While the latter studies have indicated that in some cases there are low long-term remission rates with itraconazole, there have also been studies showing similar results for terbinafine. For instance, patients treated with 250 mg terbinafine daily for 3–6 months were followed for approximately 2.5 years. Although the status of some patients changed from 'cured' to 'not cured' and vice versa, nearly half of the patients were clinically cured after 1 year and had clinical and mycological cure at 2.5 years.[7]

Reasons for prevention

These studies suggest that the long-term outlook for some patients receiving treatment for fungal nail disease is unsatisfactory because of treatment failure, relapse or re-infection.[8]

Failure of treatment of onychomycosis may be due to re-infection or to incomplete eradication of the original fungus by treatment (relapse) (see Table 7.10), although in most cases it is virtually impossible to distinguish re-infections from true relapses. Failures that occur within 1 year after interruption of treatment are more likely to be recurrences following recrudescence of the pre-existing infection, whereas failures that occur later are probably reinfections (new infections). The latter should account for about two-thirds of relapses.[2] So, why are patients with onychomycosis so easily re-infected? Susceptibility to onychomycosis depends on several factors, including genetic predisposition, reduced nail growth rate and underlying disease.

Genetic predisposition

Trichophyton rubrum onychomycosis frequently occurs in several members of the same family in different generations (Figure 8.1). *Trichophyton rubrum* infection, however, is rare in persons marrying into infected families, suggesting a genetic predisposition rather than an intrafamilial transmission of the infection. It is associated with atopy, for instance.[9] Pedigree studies suggest an autosomal dominant inheritance.[10] According to Zaias et al.,[10] predisposed individuals acquire *T. rubrum* infection in early childhood from their infected parents. The infection remains localized to the plantar region for many years without being noticed by the patient. Nail invasion, which usually begins in adult life, is possibly favoured by local factors such as reduced nail growth rate and trauma. Genetic predisposition to *T.*

rubrum invasion may possibly be linked to biochemical abnormalities in the keratins. A genetic susceptibility to infection by *T. concentricum* (tinea imbricata) has also been suggested. In neither case have modern genetic techniques been applied to investigate the problem.

Gender has a role in determining the risk that an individual will develop onychomycosis.[11,12] In one survey, the odds of males having onychomycosis were 84.3% greater than females of the same age.[11]

Reduced nail growth rate

It has been suggested that onychomycosis affects the toenails of elderly individuals because of slow growth rate,[13] a hypothesis which is still debatable. However, the association between onychomycosis and ageing is very well established and the prevalence of the disease is expected to increase in the coming decades due to the increasing longevity of the human population.

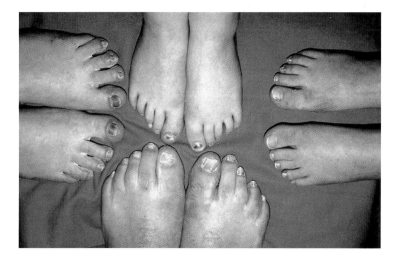

Figure 8.1

Genetic predisposition to *T. rubrum*. (Image courtesy of D.T. Roberts, UK.)

Underlying disease

Nail diseases

Onycholysis and nail bed hyperkeratosis may favour nail invasion by fungi. This explains why onychomycosis is quite common in patients with traumatic nail dystrophies or nail bed psoriasis. Onychomycosis is more common in patients with psoriasis with a prevalence ranging from 13% to 21.5%. It has been shown that psoriasis increases by 50% the risk of developing onychomycosis.[14,15]

Dermatological diseases

Dermatophyte infection is often observed in patients with palmoplantar keratoderma or ichthyosis.[16,17]

Systemic disease

Peripheral vascular disorders and diabetes mellitus have frequently been reported to predispose to onychomycosis. The association between onychomycosis and diabetes has been confirmed by several studies and we can assume that diabetics are three times more susceptible to onychomycosis than non-diabectis.[18,19]

Immunosuppression clearly predisposes to onychomycosis, and nail invasion by *Candida* is almost exclusively seen in patients with impaired immune function.

Patients with HIV infection are more commonly affected by onychomycosis than healthy individuals.[20] Predisposing factors among HIV positive patients include low CD4 count, familial history of onychomycosis, personal history of tinea pedis and walking barefoot around swimming pools.[21]

Other diseases which have been associated with onychomycosis include Cushing's syndrome,[22] peripheral neuropathies, lymphoma,[23] atopic disorders, cancer, rheumatoid disorders and gastrointestinal disorders.[24]

In some cases nail infection may represent the portal of entry for a disseminated infection. Proximal subungual onychomycosis due to *T. rubrum* is often observed in HIV patients, where it is considered to be a negative prognostic feature. For this reason, patients with *T. rubrum* proximal subungual onychomycosis should be examined for the presence of underlying immunosuppression.

Cigarette smoking

Cigarette smoking has also been found to increase the risk of developing onychomycosis.[25]

Prevention

Since relapses of onychomycosis are frequent, consideration should be given to prevention of recurrences in patients who have been cured. High rates of infections have been associated with working conditions where:

- Workers are required to wear heavy duty shoes or are exposed to wet conditions which create a confined, damp and warm atmosphere that facilitates the development of fungal and bacterial infection.
- Industries which do not provide sufficient information to workers about the importance of foot hygiene.

- Jobs which necessitate the use of communal showers, which can lead to recurrent fungal contamination.

Collective preventive measures

These are generally ineffective because they are difficult to apply and/or not adhered to.

Ideally the following situations are desirable:[26]

- Tiled shower floors should be inclined to allow sufficient drainage and non-stagnation of wastewater (*T. rubrum* survives for 25 days in stagnant water at 23–25°C).
- Wooden shower-floor grids should be replaced by plastic ones to limit the adhesion of scales shed by infected feet.
- Floors of communal showers must be washed and disinfected at least once daily with for example, sodium hypochlorite, if possible after use by each group of workers.

Individual preventive measures, have to be added to the collective preventive measures.

There is no evidence that disinfecting shoes and socks, though logical, affects the course or relapse rate of onychomycosis. However, it is important to treat recurrent tinea pedis at the earliest opportunity. In individuals at risk for tinea pedis (Table 8.1) it is important to limit spread in shower rooms by providing disposable slippers and by careful foot hygiene including drying web spaces after showering.

TABLE 8.1	Individuals at risk

Armed forces, police
Athletes
Dustmen
Employees of indoor swimming pools
Excavation workers
Mine workers
Nuclear fuel workers
Rubber-industry workers
Sewer workers
Steel and furnace workers
Wood-cutters

Tolnaftate,[27] fenticonazole,[28] ciclopiroxolamine and bifonazole powder[29] have all been used prophylactically to prevent recurrent tinea pedis. A weekly application of terbinafine cream in the nail area,[30] between the toes and on the soles of the feet would also be expected to be very effective in preventing re-infection in those individuals who appear to be particularly susceptible to onychomycosis.

Finally, long-term intermittent therapy might prevent the re-establishment of tinea pedis and limit the risk of nail re-infection. Periodic use of transungual antifungal drug delivery systems, which are retained in nail keratin after discontinuation of therapy, appears to be a logical and safe method for preventing recurrences, but this needs confirmation in a large population. However, it is doubtful if such approaches are practicable in the majority of patients and good foot hygiene at home or in the work place coupled with early treatment of recurrent tinea pedis may provide the best solution.

References

1. De Cuyper C. Long-term evaluation of terbinafine 250 and 500 mg daily in a 16-week oral treatment for toenail onychomycosis. Br J Dermatol 1996; 135:156

2. De Baker M, De Vroey C, Lesaffre E et al. Twelve weeks of continuous oral therapy for toenail onychomycosis caused by dermatophytes: a double-blind comparative trial of terbinafine 250 mg/day, versus itraconazole 200 mg/day. J Am Acad Dermatol 1998; 38:S57–S63

3. Bräutigam M. Terbinafine versus itraconazole: a controlled clinical comparison in onychomycosis of the toenails. J Am Acad Dermatol 1998; 38:S53–S56

4. Tosti A, Piraccini BM, Stinchi C et al. Relapses of onychomycosis after successful treatment with systemic antifungals: a three year follow-up. Dermatology 1998; 197:162–6

5. De Backer M, De Vroey C, Lesaffre E et al. Twelve weeks of continuous oral therapy for toenail onychomycosis caused by dermatophytes: a double-blind comparative trial of terbinafine 250 mg/day versus itraconazole 200 mg/day. J Am Acad Dermatol 1998; 38:S57–63

6. Heikkilä H, Stubb S. Long-term results of patients with onychomycosis treated with itraconazole. Acta Derm Venereol 1997; 77:70–71

7. Brandrup F, Larsen PO. Long-term follow-up of toe-nail onychomycosis treated with terbinafine. Acta Derm Venereol 1997; 77:238

8. Scher RK, Baran R. Onychomycosis in clinical practice: factors contributing to recurrence. Br J Dermatol 2003; 149 S65:5–9

9. Hanifin JM, Ray LF, Lobtiz WC. Immunological reactivity in dermatophytosis. Br J Dermatol 1974; 90:1–8

10. Zaias N, Tosti A, Rebell G et al. Autosomal dominant pattern of distal subungual onychomycosis caused by *Trichophyton rubrum*. J Am Acad Dermatol 1996; 34:302–4

11. Gupta AK, Jain HC, Lynd CW et al. Prevalence and epidemiology of unsuspected onychomycosis in patients visiting dermatologists offices in Ontario, Canada. A multicenter survey of 2001 patients. Int J Dermatol 1998; 36:783–7

12. Elewski BE, Charif MA. Prevalence of onychomycosis in patients attending a dermatology clinic in northeastern Ohio for other conditions. Arch Dermatol 1997; 133:1172–3

13. Orentreich N, Markofsky JV, Ogelman JH. The effect of aging on the rate of linear nail growth. J Invest Dermatol 1979; 73:126–30

14. Gupta AK, Lynde CQ, Jain HC et al. A higher prevalence of onychomycosis in psoriatics compared with non-psoriatics: a multicentre study. Br J Dermatol 1997; 136:786

15. Larsen GK, Haedersdal M, Sveigaard EL. The prevalence of onychomycosis in patients with psoriasis and other skin diseases. Acta Derm Venereol 2003; 83:206–9

16. Nielsen PG, Faergemann J. Dermatophytes and keratin in patients with hereditary palmoplantar keratoderma. Acta Derm Venereol 1993; 73:416–18

17. Hay RJ. Chronic dermatophyte infections. Clinical and mycological features. Br J Dermatol 1982; 106:1–7

18. Gupta AK, Konnikov N, MacDonald P et al. Prevalance and epidemiology of toenail onychomycosis in diabetic subject: a multicentre survey. Br J Dermatol 1998; 139:665–71

19. Dogra S, Kumar B, Bhansali A, Chakrabarty A. Epidemiology of onychomycosis in patients with diabetes mellitus in India. Int J Dermatol 2002; 41:647–51

20. Daniel III CR, Norton LA, Scher RK. The spectrum of nail disease in patients with human immunodeficiency virus infection. J Am Acad Dermatol 1992; 27:93–9

21. Gupta AK, Taborda P, Taborda V et al. Epidemiolgy and prevalence of onychomycosis in HIV-positive individuals. In J Dermatol 2000; 39:746–53

22. Nelson LM, Mc Niece KJ. Recurrent Cushing's syndrome with *Trichophyton*

rubrum infection. Arch Dermatol 1959;
80:700–4

23. Lewis GM, Hopper ME, Scott MJ.
Generalised *Trichophyton rubrum* infection
associated with systemic lymphoblastoma.
Arch Derm 1953; 67:247–62

24. Sigurgeirsson B, Steingrimsson O. Risk
factors associated with onychomycosis. J Eur
Acad Dermatol Venereol. 2004; 18:48–51

25. Gupta AK, Gupta MA, Summerbell RC et al.
The epidemiology of onychomycosis:
possible role of smoking and peripheral
arterial disease. J Eur Acad Dermatol
Venereol. 2000; 14:466–9

26. Baran R. Onychomycosis. In Grob JJ, Stern
RS, MacKie RM, Weinstock WA, eds

27. Smith EB, Dickson JE, Knox JM. Tolnafate
powder in prophylaxis of tinea pedis. South
Med J 1974; 67:776–8

28. Albanese G, Cintio R, Giorgetti P et al.
Recurrent tinea pedis: a double blind study
on the prophylactic use of fenticonazole
powder. Mycoses 1992; 35:157–9

29. Galimberti RL, Belli L, Negroni R et al.
Prophylaxis of tinea pedis interdigitalis with
bifonazole. 1% powder. Dermatologica 1984;
169 Suppl 1:111–16

30. Evans EG, Seaman RA, James IG.
Short-duration therapy with terbinafine
1% cream in dermatophyte skin infections.
Br J Dermatol 1994; 130:83–7

Epidemiology, Causes and Prevention of
Skin Diseases. Oxford, Blackwell, 1997:276–8

Index